Critical Realism for Welfare Professions

T0270849

As a discipline, social work needs an inclusive metatheory for both research and practice that goes beyond positivism and constructivism. This is the first book to present and discuss how critical realism can contribute to a more useful and realistic approach to both research and practice in social work. As a theory of science that includes normative theories and emphasises method-pluralism and holistic thinking, critical realism is applicable to a world of poverty, global health problems and social conflicts.

Contributors to this book present a realist perspective on social work. The connection between critical realism and social work is illuminated through a theoretical introduction in Part 1. Part 2 covers the specific topics of normativity, interdisciplinarity and education. Part 3 presents practical/empirical examples from contemporary research in social work, using different approaches based on critical realism.

As critical realism can contribute to a useful and realistic approach to research and practice, this book is essential reading for professionals, academics and students working in different fields of social work and health care.

Monica Kjørstad is Associate Professor in Social Work at the Faculty of Social Sciences at Oslo and Akershus University College of Applied Sciences. Her interests are social administration and planning, leadership and implementation issues connected to social work, welfare and human rights. She holds a PhD in social work and social policy.

May-Britt Solem is Associate Professor in Social Work at the Faculty of Social Sciences at Oslo and Akershus University College of Applied Sciences. She has constructed and now coordinates the Master Program in Family Therapy. Her current research is a longitudinal study of parenting practices and stress and sons' transitions to adulthood. She holds a PhD in psychology.

Routledge Advances in Social Work

www.routledge.com/Routledge-Advances-in-Social-Work/book-series/RASW

Critical Realism for Welfare Professions

Edited by Monica Kjørstad
and May-Britt Solem

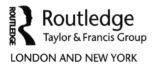

LONDON AND NEW YORK

First published 2018 by Routledge

2 Park Square, Milton Park, Abingdon, Oxfordshire OX14 4RN

52 Vanderbilt Avenue, New York, NY 10017

Routledge is an imprint of the Taylor & Francis Group, an informa business

First issued in paperback 2019

British Library Cataloguing-in-Publication Data
A catalogue record for this book is available from the British Library

Library of Congress Cataloging-in-Publication Data
Names: Kjørstad, Monica, editor. | Solem, May-Britt, editor.
Title: Critical realism for welfare professions / edited by Monica Kjørstad and May-Britt Solem.
Description: Abingdon, Oxon ; New York, NY : Routledge, 2017. | Series: Routledge advances in social work | Includes bibliographical references and index.
Identifiers: LCCN 2017009853 | ISBN 9781138699199 (hardback) | ISBN 9781315517537 (ebook)
Subjects: LCSH: Social service. | Social service—Practice. | Critical realism.
Classification: LCC HV40 .C727 2017 | DDC 361.3—dc23
LC record available at https://lccn.loc.gov/2017009853

ISBN: 978-1-138-69919-9 (hbk)
ISBN: 978-0-367-35241-7 (pbk)

Typeset in Times New Roman
by Apex CoVantage, LLC

Contents

Figures

Editors' preface

The intention with this book is to demonstrate the potential of critical realism as a metatheory of science for social research. As teachers and researchers in social and welfare work and family therapy, we shared a common interest searching for an integrative theory in our fields of research.

The work by Roy Bhaskar has been an inspiration for our book. The last time this book project was discussed with him was at the International Association of Critical Realism conference in London in July 2014. As always, he offered his wisdom and generosity that brought so much encouragement and consolation to fellow scholars. It was a great loss when he died in November 2014.

This book is ambitiously intended to be both an introduction to critical realism and an in-depth elaboration of some central premises for critical realism as a metatheory. The chapters from Andrew Sayer about normative issues in the social sciences, Berth Danermark on the necessity of an interdisciplinary approach in social research and Stan Houston and Lorna Montgomery about their critical realist perspectives and ideas on education are all contributions that substantiate critical realism as ontology. We are deeply grateful for these strong contributions.

The last part of this book presents different ways of using critical realism as a metatheoretical ground for empirical projects. The chapters by Harry Lunabba, Elina Pekkarinen, May-Britt Solem and Monica Kjørstad are unfolding a diverse and flourishing juxtaposition by scholars from different fields of research. They demonstrate empirically that the ontology of critical realism may be a contribution to a better understanding of our messy and chaotic world.

Finally, we wish to thank Oslo and Akershus University College of Applied Sciences for their economic support for language editing.

Oslo, 30 January 2017
The editors

Contributors

Berth Danermark is Professor of Sociology in the School of Health Sciences at Örebro University, Sweden. He is the Director of Doctoral Studies at the Swedish Institute of Disability Research. In collaboration with researchers in other disciplines, he has developed an interdisciplinary approach where a behavioral and social science perspective is interwoven technically and medically.

Stan Houston practiced social work with children and families in Northern Ireland for around twenty years before entering higher education. He is interested in the application of critical social theory and philosophy to social work.

Monica Kjørstad is Associate Professor in Social Work at the Faculty of Social Sciences at Oslo and Akershus University College of Applied Sciences. She holds a PhD in social work and social policy. Her fields of interest are social administration and planning, leadership, human rights and the theory of science. Her research interests are about implementation issues related to professional social and welfare work in the public sector. She worked as co-editor of the journal *Nordic Social Work Research* (2011–2015).

Harry Lunabba, PhD, is currently working as a Senior Lecturer at the Swedish School of Social Science, University of Helsinki, within the field of social work. He has a professional background in child protection social work. His current research interests are childhood, youth and gender studies within the context of schooling and welfare practices. His teaching focuses mainly on social work practices, ethnography and childhood studies.

Lorna Montgomery practiced as a social worker in Northern Ireland for around twenty years, mainly in the area of mental health. She is interested in the application of theory to social work, and in research around mental health, adult safeguarding and bereavement.

Elina Pekkarinen, PhD (SocSc), is a Researcher at the Finnish Youth Research Network and a Chairman of the Finnish Society for Childhood Studies. As a former social worker, she is experienced in child welfare, emergency and poverty issues. Fields of her academic interest include social work, child welfare, childhood studies, youth studies and critical realism.

Andrew Sayer is Professor of Social Theory and Political Economy at Lancaster University, UK. His current interests are inequality, ethics and social life, as elaborated in his books *The Moral Significance of Class* (Cambridge University Press, 2005) and *Why Things Matter to People: Social Science, Values and Ethical Life* (Cambridge University Press, 2011). He also works on "moral economy". His latest book – *Why We Can't Afford the Rich* (Policy Press, 2014) – develops this last theme, as does ongoing work on climate change, sustainability and economic organisation.

May-Britt Solem is Associate Professor at Oslo and Akershus University of Applied Sciences. She holds a PhD in Psychology and is responsible for, teaches and supervises in the master's program of family therapy. Solem started "Family Research Network" in Norway, and was a board member from 2003 to 2010. She was a member of the editorial board for the *International Journal of Multiple Research Approaches* from 2008 to 2013. Her present research is a longitudinal study of parents' coping practices and their sons' transitions to adulthood from a life course perspective.

Part I

1 Toward an in-depth understanding of professional social and welfare work

Monica Kjørstad and May-Britt Solem

Introduction

The overarching aim of this book is to contribute to the development of knowledge for social welfare and health work professions by bringing a critical realist perspective on fields such as social welfare, childcare, family care, health care, and social policy. Critical realism, as a theoretical position in the social sciences, is based on the understanding that reality is stratified, which means that biological, psychological, and social elements are viewed as interwoven and interdependent for people's life experiences, and quality of life. In the holistic perspectives on social work, in both a theoretical and practical sense, these three elements together are important for understanding of how one can assist people with different kinds of social and health problems. This point may be obvious, but it is also complicated. Nevertheless, investigating peoples' subjective experiences and investigating reality as stratified may contribute to a deeper understanding of practice situations. This book deals with this perspective.

From a critical realist perspective, the focus of the research process is the relation between the real world and the concepts we form of it (Danermark et al., 2002, p. 15). Reality has an objective existence (the intransitive dimension), but our knowledge about it is conceptually mediated (the transitive dimension). In summary, one could say that knowledge is theory-dependent, but not theory-determined. We also understand science as a practical activity. This book will discuss how critical realism as a theory of science may contribute to a more useful and realistic approach to both research and practice in social work.

The transitive dimension is our beliefs about what exists, and includes our knowledge of reality, while the intransitive dimension includes the generative mechanisms (the object about which science aims to acquire knowledge) that exist independently of our knowledge about them. These generative mechanisms generate events and action. Bhaskar introduced the concept of "double inclusiveness", which means that critical realism is compatible with a variety of methods and that the object of study in social work research constructs the direction and choice of methods (Bhaskar & Danermark, 2006). Critical realism includes insights from other metatheoretical perspectives without reducing our understanding to either positivist or constructivist positions; to a view of the world that ontologically goes further to include multiple domains of reality – the empirical, actual, and real (Bhaskar & Danermark, 2006). Social work needs a more inclusive metatheory for both research and practice that goes beyond positivism and constructivism. This metatheory includes normative assessments in professional social work practice, and because of this inclusiveness, professional actions and interactions to perform liberation and emancipation of people become evident.

Consequently, critical realism emphasizes method-pluralism and holistic thinking, and includes normative theories that are applicable to a world that suffers from poverty, health problems, and social conflict (Houston, 2001a). The aim of the present book is to focus on these dynamic relations by presenting examples of research studies using a critical realism perspective. We will also illuminate practical situations in which critical realism may be tools for individual or family counseling and clinical practice. First, social work does indeed have an emancipatory agenda. Normative assessments, decisions, and interventions are conducted in *all* practice situations. By assisting individuals and families in difficult life situations, social work addresses social injustices and promotes social change.

The emancipatory agenda

In the fourth ethical dimension in his dialectics, Bhaskar developed a complex scheme of ethical elements involving, in bare terms, what it means to be free, to trust, and to enter into relations of solidarity with others. He discussed the principles of dialectical rationality that press human beings, through the necessary universalization of their practical commitments, toward ethical positions. Bhaskar used the concept of "ethical agency" (Bhaskar, 1993).

Archer (1995; 2000) claims that critical realism advances human capacity to influence structure and bring about change in our own lives. Archer (1995; 2007) also argues that critical realism provides more than just breadth, depth, and a focus on structure by stating that critical realism advances human capacity to influence structure, conditions that construct suffering, and difficult life situations. Human agency has the capacity to "overcome and even change these structures" (Brian-Lawson, 2012, p. 524).

It is important for all welfare professions to have a thorough understanding of the relationship between economic and political structures and ideological patterns that impede a person or a group from addressing unjust social systems. However, in addition to understanding, it is essential to have tools for action. Therefore, social research should have a liberating function and an emancipatory agenda. In practical social work, salutogenic or health-promoting thinking goes together with an actor perspective that involves empowerment and/or emancipatory practice. Professionals working in the health and welfare sector disclose social problems and social injustice that influence people's quality of life (Collins et al., 2010).

One task of the social scientist is to understand the interconnection between human agency and a social structure that exhibits causal powers within a temporal and spatial context (Houston, 2010). For example, social work is an applied discipline; it is 'relational' and value-driven, which means that the theories must be applicable to practice situations. The following definition was approved by the International Federation of Social Work (IFSW) and the International Association of Schools of Social Work (IASSW) at IFSW's General Assembly in Melbourne, Australia, in July 2014:

> Social work is a practice-based profession and an academic discipline that promotes social change and development, social cohesion, and the empowerment and liberation of people. Principles of social justice, human rights, collective responsibility and respect for diversities are central to social work. Underpinned by theories of social work, social sciences, humanities and indigenous knowledge, social work engages people and structures to address life challenges and enhance wellbeing. The above definition may be amplified at national and/or regional levels.

This definition emphasizes that professional social and welfare work is an academic discipline that has its basis in professional practice. The definition also notes that professional social work is a normative activity in which social justice and human rights are fundamental entities. The society should act as a sort of guarantor for collective responsibilities for people's well-being, which means that human rights need to coexist alongside collective responsibility. The IFSW comments to the core-mandates underline that social work is based on holistic biopsychosocial, spiritual assessments and that interventions that transcend the micro-macro divide, incorporating multiple system levels and inter-sectorial and inter-professional collaboration are aimed at sustainable development. Social change, liberation, and emancipation are key concepts in social work. This definition of social work leads to the relevance of critical realism as a social theory that has the potential to include the theoretical and practical sides of social work as an academic discipline.

Theory, practice, and the intellectual fallacy

The importance of professional social and welfare work as a theoretical discipline and research area has often been questioned, with one of the main objections being that social work is strongly identified with practice, not with theory (Levin, 2004). In recent years, however, it has been argued that practical knowledge has gradually lost its place in social and welfare work and some scholars have maintained that there is a knowledge crisis (Longhofer & Floresch, 2012; Göppner, 2012; Houston, 2012). However, we will argue that if there is a knowledge crisis, this must be solved by again accepting practical knowledge as a grounded position in professional social and welfare work. Andrew Sayer (1997) has argued that some extreme representatives of a social constructivist position have missed the important point that some things have more of an essence than others. He claims that theorizing without any reference to praxis is an "intellectual fallacy" and criticises the belief "that knowledge is gained purely through contemplation or observation of the world" (Sayer, 1992, p. 13). Praxis (reality) is characterized by its complexity, and when people are in difficult life situations, social workers are expected to help to elucidate those complex problems. Social work must be recognized as a legitimate knowledge-producing discipline within the academic (McLaughlin, 2012). We argue that it is important to contribute to relationship-based practice knowledge and to critical understanding of practical evidence-based work.

The contemporary discourses often still have a perceptible gap between theory and practice. Although many professionals might argue that the unit of analysis in social and welfare work is the "person in the situation" or the "individual in society", it seems difficult to take the implications of this into thorough consideration. Nevertheless, different user participation strategies such as empowerment practices, health promotion perspectives (coping and resilience), citizenship theories, and human rights perspectives are examples of new paradigms where the structure – agency relation – is very much in focus. An increasing focus on public health in general may indeed force professional social and welfare workers to view health-related issues more broadly. As a part of public health work, we understand the aim of professional work in the social and welfare sector to be to help people reduce health and social risks factors and to strengthen the protective factors that contribute to better health (Solem, 2013).

One of the challenges for social work is to integrate a balanced person-in-environment perspective and to go beyond the sociocultural focus that places minimal emphasis on the individual. At the same time, we must move beyond the individual focus, which does not pay a great deal of attention to the environment. Social work as a discipline needs more than one analytic perspective to catch the complexity in practice. This is particularly important when analyzing a certain context to find underlying mechanisms that influence phenomena such as different policy implementation processes and their consequences. This is what a critical realist approach should do. In doing so, we may be able to go under the surface and, as Stan Houston put it, return to depth in social work practice (Houston, 2001a). This may be achieved using different pluralistic methodological approaches and by studying the phenomena at several levels: societal, institutional, and individual. Such an approach makes it possible to shed light on the connection between the different levels of these phenomena. The approach begins by acknowledging that the phenomena under study are *real*, but that they are not always manifestly disclosed.

Reality: historically and contextually contingent

From our point of view, critical realism may offer an alternative to the relativism inherent within social constructionism. Consequently, critical realism may be an alternative to the incomplete positions of positivism and constructivism, each of which offers conflation of the ontological and epistemological questions.

For example, in order to more clearly understand a family with a child who is struggling with mental health problems, various mechanisms at the biological, psychological, social, and cultural levels need to be investigated.

Some representatives of a constructionist view on society sometimes argue against the notion that there are essential structures within the society or the individual. For example, it is important to note that diagnoses are reductionist categorizations that are socially constructed. They represent selected snap-shots of unique children at special times when the problems appear serious enough to be investigated further (Hertz, 2008). Nevertheless, many of these children suffer and become stigmatized because their problems are viewed as being caused only by the child. According to Hacking (2000), behavioral problems are an example of an interactive category because this category itself may influence those who are placed in it. Hacking also argued the importance of being aware of what categorizations do to individuals who become trapped in them.

Evidence-based knowledge – evidence-based practice

Social science phenomena are characterized by complexity, by their dependence on context, and by the interplay between several motivating forces. This involves theoretical and methodological challenges. In order for knowledge to be appli-cable, we must first assume that we are acquainted with the mechanisms that produce empirical events – that is, health and social problems – and these mecha-nisms are seldom directly observable. This implies that empirical observations alone often have limited value when explaining human action (Bhaskar, 1978; 1998; Kjørstad, 2008; Sayer, 2008).

Nevertheless, certain cause-and-effect models can provide necessary knowl-edge about the manifest effects of a particular practice. However, someone who is interested in *why* and *how* social work is able to influence a result must thoroughly investigate the situations and events in which social work is practiced and situ-ated. This strength of the critical realist perspective is in addition to, rather than instead of, other types of research perspectives. For example, there is a need to know more about why certain coping strategies are used, when they are used, and when/why they work or not (Collins et al., 2010), and also *how*.

Understanding human lives by crossing boundaries

Interdisciplinary research crosses traditional boundaries between academic disci-plines and schools of thought. Interdisciplinary research and social work practices both investigate a common complex phenomenon and how that phenomenon is manifested at different levels of reality. The aim is to catch both the social and the psychological conditions in people's situations. Reflexive thinking or "meaning making" is a complex process that is influenced by appraisals of social support, personal characteristics, and environmental factors.

In different framings, social work aims to understand the interconnection between human agency and a social structure that exhibits causal powers within a temporal and spatial context (Houston, 2012). Because of this broad focus, social work must be viewed with an interdisciplinary approach, focusing on the relation between the individual and the environment, and between structure (living reality of the agent) and actor/agent, and these practices must be understood as process-oriented and systemic. Critical realism emphasizes interdisciplinarity and methodological pluralism in research, because of its focus on complex interplay between phenomena in social practices. In Chapter 4, Berth Danermark discusses interdisciplinarity in research, both theoretically and practically.

The normative position of social and welfare work: a strength for research?

Andrew Sayer (2011) has raised a number of fundamental questions: Why do people care about things? Why do we care about how people behave toward each other in a moral and ethical sense? Moreover, why do we care about how the world looks and is organized? If we care about our relation to the world in our daily lives, what does that mean for social science? Many people would say that the job of a social scientist is to describe, explain, and hopefully understand, but not to evaluate or judge. Sayer is arguing that values and norms are a necessary and invaluable part of life. Although social science aims to understand and explain rather than to decide how to act, we must be evaluative.

Sayer argues that any research that claims to be critical must have an opinion about the particular position or point of view from which the criticism comes. Therefore, norms and values must be scrutinized in the same way as all other kinds of explanations. A key question is whether there is a tendency to make normative questions "sociological" by insisting that specific norms and values are embedded in specific social circumstances, and must be analyzed accordingly. However, it is still crucial to have an opinion about what is good or bad. A sociological argument sometimes used *against* normative thinking is that behavior is a habit, rather than something governed by rational assessments of normative principles of morality. Therefore, according to Sayer, the social sciences often underestimate such everyday evaluation and self-reflection, interpretation, and reasoning as a natural part of ordinary life. One does not always define this consciously as ethical or normative theory, but this is the reality for professional social and welfare workers who are constantly confronted with ethical dilemmas in their daily work.

Because of this reasoning, the main argument for a normative perspective in the social sciences is the need to modify positivism's distinct separation between what *is* and what *should be*. For example, when social workers are identifying unsatisfied needs and human rights, they must make some kind of assessment of what is good and what is desirable from a normative assessment. A critical approach implies a connection between positive (that is, explanatory and descriptive) observations and a normative social discourse based on moral and political philosophy. In Chapter 3, Andrew Sayer discusses normativity in the social sciences in greater depth.

Content and structure of the book

The book is structured in four parts. In the Part I and Chapter 1 of the book, "Toward an in-depth understanding of professional social and welfare work", Monica Kjørstad and May-Britt Solem present an introduction to the book followed by "Basic concepts in critical realism" in Chapter 2.

In Chapter 3 in Part II of the book, Andrew Sayer discusses the nature of normativity in life, including professional work, and how the social sciences can contribute to a better understanding of this. In this chapter, entitled "Normativity in the social sciences and professions", Sayer argues that social science has been handicapped by inadequate views of values as merely subjective or conventional, and by assumptions that facts and values are radically distinct. In contrast, it is proposed that normativity and values need to be understood as fundamentally concerned with well-being, and that this is not simply culturally relative. In keeping with critical realism, but also Aristotelianism and the ethic of care, a view of ethics is proposed in which attentiveness to the specificities of the other, rather than compliance with general norms, is the central feature. This position is elaborated in relation to care and dignity and finally, the problems of post-structuralist social science's hostility to normativity are criticised.

In Chapter 4, Berth Danermark treats interdisciplinarity in a broad sense (a biopsychosocial approach), comprising a number of disciplines or professions. He introduces the concept of "necessarily laminated systems" as an integrative analytical tool for investigating complex phenomenon. Professionals and researchers constantly encounter complex problems. To address them in an interdisciplinary manner, by putting interdisciplinarity into practice, is a demanding task. Interdisciplinarity is a natural consequence of the open-systemic character within which practically all events occur. The aim of the chapter is to elaborate the challenging process of interdisciplinary work. In the course of the chapter, the author describes the pertinent features of four phases of the interdisciplinarity process. The chapter would be especially relevant for those who are concerned with interdisciplinarity in the field of health and social work: professionals, consultants, researchers and the clients.

In Chapter 5 by Stan Houston and Lorna Montgomery entitled "Learning to *absent* the absent: critical realism and social work", the authors are arguing that social work is continuously extending its explanatory reach by drawing on theories from the social sciences. In particular, the field of metatheory is beginning to ignite scholarly interest. Regarding the latter, some commentators have highlighted how critical realism can assist the profession to apprehend the deep-seated causes of behaviour and of human oppression. However, how to convey the schematic and abstract nature of critical realism to social workers presents a challenge. The chapter addresses this necessity by arguing that problem-based learning presents a model of inquiry that enables students to grasp and apply critical realism's core tenets to practical concerns in the social world. In doing so, it enables them to respond to human oppression in a more insightful way.

Part III of the book consists of four contributions presenting various empirical research projects. The intention of this part of the book is to show how critical realism can be applied in different ways, often combined with other theories and methodologies of social sciences. The shared ontological approach is critical realism.

The first chapter (Chapter 6) in Part III of the book, written by Monica Kjørstad, presents a discussion of how a critical realist approach can be used as an analytical tool to understand the dynamics among social politics, institutions of social welfare, and professional social and welfare implementation work. The discussion is illustrated by an empirical project about implementation of a workfare policy in Norway as an example. Conclusively, Kjørstad argues that the critical realist approach made it possible to uncover and understand the dialectic relation between the body of law and existing policies, institutional practices, and the practice of social workers.

In Chapter 7, Harry Lunabba discusses the implementation of critical realist theory when conducting ethnographic research. The chapter is entitled "Encounters uncovered – implementing critical realism and domain theory in ethnographic research with young masculinities". The foundational idea of the chapter is that critical realist theory offers concepts of how to manage and make sense of complex ethnographic data.

In Chapter 8, May-Britt Solem presents her research project within the field of family therapy, entitled "Parenting stress and coping practices in a critical realist perspective". Her analytical focus was to examine parenting as situated practices, and whether there were differences between a clinical and a comparison group regarding parental conditions in parenting practices. Another aim was to explore predictors to parenting stress as family demographics, child's behaviour problems, parents' resources and capacities. The results revealed mechanisms in play influencing parenting stress in the parenting situations.

In Chapter 9, Elina Pekkarinen presents her project "Positions of young people in child welfare – 'TMSA' in research practice". Her article describes how the application of Roy Bhaskar's Transformational Model of Social Activity (TMSA) and its position-practice system, function as a metatheoretical framework in empirical social work research that applies theoretical concepts from the theory of societal reaction. By representing a unique position model, it demonstrates step by step how this critical realist framework may be applied to a qualitative study outlining the experiences of eight young people that have been placed into out-of-home care by a child welfare agency.

Finally, Monica Kjørstad and May-Britt Solem conclude this project in the last chapter (Part IV, Chapter 10) under the heading "Theory and practice as a dynamic relation".

References

Archer, M. S. (1995) *Realist Social Theory: The Morphogenetic Approach*, Cambridge: Cambridge University Press.

Archer, M. S. (2000) *Being Human: The Problem of Agency*, Cambridge: Cambridge University Press.

Archer, M. S. (2007) *Making Our Way Through the World*, Cambridge: Cambridge University Press.

Bhaskar, R. (1978) *A Realist Theory of Science*, Brighton: Harvester Press.

Bhaskar, R. (1993) *Dialectic: The Pulse of Freedom*, London: Verso.

Bhaskar, R. (1998) *The Possibility of Naturalism*, London: Routledge.

Bhaskar, R., & Danermark, B. (2006) Metatheory, interdisciplinarity and disability research – A critical realist perspective, *Scandinavian Journal of Disability Research*, 4, 278–297.

Brian-Lawson, K. (2012) Response: Critical realism: Response to Longhofer and Floresch, *Research on Social Work Practice*, 22(5), 523–528, doi:10.1177/1049731512454015.

Collins, K. M. T., Onwuegbuzie, A. J., & Jiao, Q. G. (2010) *Toward a Broaderunderstanding of Stress and Coping: Mixed Methods Approaches*, Charlotte, NC: Information Age Publishing.

Danermark, B., Ekström, M., Jakobsen, L., & Karlsson, J. C. (2002) *Explaining Society: Critical Realism in the Social Sciences*, London: Routledge.

Göppner, H. J. (2012) Response: Epistyemological issues of social work science as a transactional action science, *Research on Social Work Practice*, 22(5), 542–547, doi:101177/1049731512442250.

Hacking, I. (2000) *Social Construction of What?* Stockholm, Sweden: Thales.

Hertz, S. (2008) *Børne-og ungdomspsykiatri: Nye perspektiver og uanede muligheter* [Child and Adolescent Psychiatry: New Perspectives and Unexpected Possibilities], Copenhagen, Denmark: Akademisk Forlag.

Houston, S. (2001a) Beyond social constructionism: Critical realism and social work, *British Journal of Social Work*, 31, 845–861.

Houston, S. (2010) Prising open the black box: CR, action research and social work, *Qualitative Social Work*, 9, 73–91.

Houston, S. (2012) Response: Reviewing the coming crisis in social work: A response to Longhofer and Floersch, *Research on Social Work Practice*, 22(5), 520–522, doi:10.1177/1049731512441264.

Kjørstad, M. (2008) Opening the black box – Mobilizing practical knowledge in social research: Methodological reflections based on a study of social work practice, *Qualitative Social Work*, 7(2), 143–161.

Levin, I. (2004) Living Apart Together: A New Family Form. In Rosenheil, S. & Budgeon, S. (eds.), *Beyond the Conventional Family: Cares, Intimacy and Community in the 21st Century*, London: Sage, pp. 223–240.

Longhofer, J., & Floersch, J. (2012) The coming crisis in social work: Some thoughts on social work and science, *Research on Social Work Practice*, 22(5), 499–519, doi:10.1177/1049731512445509.

McLaughlin, H. (2012) *Understanding Social Work Research*, London: Sage.

Sayer, A. (1992) *Method in Social Science: A Realist Approach*, London: Routledge.

Sayer, A. (1997) Essentialism, social constructionism, and beyond, *The Sociological Review*, 45, 453–487.

Sayer, A. (2008) *Realism and Social Science*, London: Sage.
Sayer, A. (2011) *Why Things Matter to People: Social Science, Values and Ethical Life*, Cambridge: Cambridge University Press.
Solem, M. B. (2013) Understanding parenting as situated in the larger sociocultural context in clinical social work, *Child and Adolescent Social Work Journal*, 30(1), 61–78, doi:10.1007/s10560-012-0278-9.

2 Basic concepts in critical realism

Monica Kjørstad and May-Britt Solem

Introduction

This chapter presents the basic concepts of critical realism. We understand critical realism as a holistic theory of science, and as a dynamic relation between human agency and structure. Through examples, we illustrate how critical realism as a social theory may have strong relevance for professions working in the social and welfare sector. We draw a short historical line to the development of critical realism and introduce the ontology and epistemology of critical realism. We also present our understanding of reality as stratified and discuss generative mechanisms that are at work in open social systems. Finally, we explain and discuss a central construct: the emergence and emergent powers. Through examples, we show how emergent (powerful) situations appear at different levels and at different times in our day-to-day lives.

Critical theory – critical realism

A common statement is that critical theory is relatively new; that it appeared with the Frankfurt School in the mid- and late 20th century. However, this is not the case. In fact, we must go back to the Enlightenment period and long before that; early social theory had indeed the intention of being critical of the social phenomena it studied. Andrew Sayer argued that it was the fragmentation of social science disciplines that caused it to differ from the philosophy of science in the late 19th and early 20th centuries and diminished its critical element (Sayer, 2008).

The Frankfurt School was established in 1930 with the founding of the Institut für Sozialforschung in Frankfurt am Main. The characteristics of the social sciences that were developed in the Frankfurt School were the close correlation between theoretical comprehensive analyses and specific analyses oriented toward social phenomena. The connection between theoretical understanding and political practice and the strong interdependency between science and politics was evident (Kalleberg, 1992). Consequently, the Frankfurt School scientists undertook systematic analyses of the political situation to maintain a close connection between theory and practice.

At that time, a common critique from the representatives of the Frankfurt School was that traditional positivist theories had the natural sciences as their model and perceived themselves as independent of all societal interests. Jürgen Habermas followed up this critique, but in a different and extended way, arguing that a new interpretation of science in society was needed.

Critical realism was articulated in the 1970s and shares some of the same basic understandings of the relationships among science, society, and politics that are found in the Frankfurt School. Similarities may be found with respect to the development of social work as a profession. A common argument is that the ambiguity that is sometimes found in social work practices has much to do with its close connection to political and moral activities. Professionals working in the social and welfare sector should intervene in situations where the question of personal freedom, conflicts, interests, and different lifestyles and life projects must be handled in situations where there is always a lack of financial resources.

Reinventing ontology in social research

Steve Fleetwood (2004) has argued that the term ontology refers to the study or theory of being, not to being itself. To have an ontology is to have a *theory* of what exists. From our point of view, one may say that social work's ontology is about how we understand peoples' "being", not how they live their lives. Thus, one could claim that there are different types of ontologies. This is important because one may recognize the discussions and schisms in social work that concern, among other things, whether one should direct one's interventions toward the *individual* or the *environment*, or both; this is about a theory of *being* (Fleetwood & Ackroyd, 2004).

Critical realism builds upon the assumption that reality is external and independent, at the same time as being socially and historically constructed (Danermark et al., 2002; Morén & Blom, 2003). If we can avoid the mistaken epistemological conclusion – that is, if we can avoid reducing questions about *being* to questions of *how we can know* – we can recognize that knowledge has two dimensions: an intransitive one and a transitive one (Bhaskar, 1986; Sayer, 2008). It is also assumed that there is a level of reality that cannot be observed directly. However, this level can still be studied, and knowledge of this level can be collected by utilizing conceptualizations and theoretical work (for example, by interpreting empirical observations). At this level, one can discover the forces and mechanisms that produce effects. In this way, one may become able to make the potential for change in social phenomena comprehensible, in addition to searching for external causal factors (Morén & Blom, 2003). For example, when social workers deal with social injustice in action research, the research team may focus both on dialogues with the clients and with investigating mechanisms in play, which may cause a difficult (emergent) life situation for them.

A critical realist understanding ensures that it does not reduce ontology to epistemology. Roy Bhaskar calls this the *epistemological fallacy*, by which he means that it is a mistake to believe that questions of being can always be reduced to questions of knowledge or to discourses about being. The reverse is called the *ontological fallacy*, or the tendency to reduce questions of knowledge to questions of being; that is, the idea that reality can be read, known, or grasped directly – that the transitive dimension can, in some way, be dissolved (Archer et al., 1998).

Examining these distinctions may make it easier to understand why critical realism places itself as an alternative to empirical realism, on the one hand, and as an alternative to an extreme constructivist position on the other. A clear distinction is made between being and knowledge about being, with *being* given priority. This brings us to the understanding of reality.

Understanding reality as stratified

What distinguishes critical realism from other forms of realism is an understanding that reality is divided into three domains (Bhaskar, 1978).

First, there is the *empirical domain*, which consists of our experiences and observations. The second domain is the *factual domain*, which consists of all the phenomena and situations that appear, regardless of whether we are aware of them or not. Those two domains are the traditional empirical level, which is far from enough for understanding social phenomena and is definitely not sufficient for understanding why and how social problems appear. This is why the third domain is particularly important. The third domain is the *real domain* that consists of all the structurers and mechanisms that are not always observable. These structures and mechanisms, under certain circumstances, support and sometimes cause the situations and practical events within the factual domain (see Figure 2.1; Bhaskar 1978; Sayer 2000).

The three domains cannot be reduced according to each other; this represents an understanding of causality that is very different from causality based on empirical regularities. A critical realist understanding is that reality consists of open systems, which means that your understanding is based on a multi-causal view of the world.

Domains	Contents
The empirical	*Experiences and observations*
The factual	*Phenomena and situations*
The real	*Structures, mechanisms, causal potentials, and tendencies*

Figure 2.1 Three domains of reality

Sources: Bhaskar (1978); Sayer (2000).

Life is lived in open systems

One of the central questions within critical realism was formulated by the philosopher of science, Roy Bhaskar. He asked: *How can reality be so constituted that phenomena like regularity and laws can appear?* The answer is that these qualities presuppose "closed conditions" (Bhaskar, 1986). Problems connected to prediction in the social sciences are tied to the unpredictability of human judgments and choices.

In *system theory*, an open system is one that continuously interacts with its environment or surroundings. An open system interacts and interfaces by receiving inputs from and delivering outputs to the outside. In the social sciences, an open system is a process that exchanges material, energy, people, capital, and information with its environment.

Because the social world is an open system, more than one mechanism will operate at any one time. Therefore, causal mechanisms must be analyzed as "tendencies". People's actions are influenced by innate psychological mechanisms as well as wider social mechanisms (Houston, 2001). Within a critical realism framework, both qualitative and quantitative methodologies are seen as appropriate for researching the underlying mechanisms that drive actions and events (Krauss, 2005). The realist paradigm is seen as a "middle ground" between poles of positivism and constructivism (Krauss, 2005).

The dynamic relationship between human agency and structure

We have argued that social work has a close relationship to practice. We have also argued that practice needs to be reinvented with a stronger position in social work. We believe that critical realism may offer an alternative philosophical framework to the positions of positivism and constructivism for the exploration of social work issues. Critical realism examines how human agency (meanings, understandings, reasons, and intentions) interacts with the effects of social structures (social rules, norms, and laws) (Houston, 2012). In social work, in particular, we need to comprehend these two spheres to understand social life and people in difficult life situations. Social structures are real and actors do their meaning making when confronted by these structures (Houston, 2012).

Critical realism attempts to manage the problem regarding structures and actors by describing the relationship between them over time. This is in contrast to deconstructivists who find it adequate to go beyond this dimension by deconstruction, as a clearly defined methodology. Critical realism involves a holistic perspective that includes both structures and actors' interactions and theory pluralism. The structures are reproduced through intentional individual actions. If many actors change their patterns of actions, this will, over time, result in altered structures. Structures have an independent existence, which means that society must be perceived as comprising individuals, intentional individuals, *and* under-lying structures and mechanisms (Bhaskar, 1986). Archer (2000; 2003) warns that the individual is reduced to the social. There is no clear way of understand-ing how human actions engage in the world. She argues that human agency has the capacity to "overcome and even change these structures" (Brian-Lawson, 2012, p. 524).

Generative mechanisms at play in open systems

One motivation behind the development of mechanism explanations in social work is dissatisfaction with the traditional approaches toward linear causal expla-nations of events and situations with a high degree of complexity.

Critical realism emphasizes the search for basic conditions; that is, mecha-nisms that constitute the phenomenon being studied. In this way, critical realism differs from empiricism. However, both empiricism and critical realism assume that reality exists independently of the observer, although empiricism assumes that knowledge of reality is directly based on detailed studies of what can be observed. Empiricism is intended to reduce the importance of the observer's role and contextual conditions, and research aims to find empirical regulari-ties in the nature of general laws. Remembering Bhaskar's question – *How can reality be so constituted that phenomena like regularity and laws can appear?* – one must try to think differently. A critical realist perspective involves a level of reality that cannot be observed directly, but one can still gain knowledge through theoretical work (for example, through interpretations of empirical observations). At this level, one can find the forces and mechanisms that pro-duce effects (Morén & Blom, 2003; Danermark et al., 2002). The effects of a generative mechanism are contextually contingent; context influences whether the mechanism is active or passive, or whether it is offset by some other mecha-nism (Morén & Blom, 2003).

The "clue" to finding the generative mechanisms is to get a picture of the causal chains or processes that explain how a particular social phenomenon was brought about. The concept of causal chain does not imply a linear view of causal pro-cesses. Because the social world is an open system, more than one mechanism will operate at any one time. Therefore, causal mechanisms must be analyzed as the "tendencies" of processes. Sayer (1992) states that a great deal of our knowl-edge that is insufficient for prediction might be valuable for guidance to practice (see Figure 2.2).

As noted, critical realism states that reality exists independently of our dis-courses and our knowledge of it, but that our social world is socially and his-torically constructed, meaningful, in flux, and open (Buch-Hansen & Nielsen, 2005). Mechanisms produce "tendencies" and direct our attention toward seek-ing to understand and explain those tendencies. In practical social work with a family, for example, a social worker will try to understand the whole situation, including the family's interactions and the everyday life with living conditions.

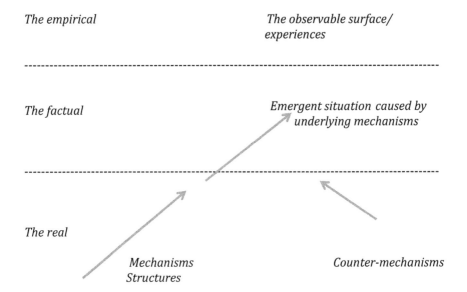

The empirical   *The observable surface/*
                                   experiences

The factual   *Emergent situation caused by*
                                   underlying mechanisms

The real

             Mechanisms   *Counter-mechanisms*
             Structures

Figure 2.2 Domains of reality and generative mechanisms at play
Source: Sayer (2000, p. 15).

An empirical correlation may not be used to identify mechanisms and does not contribute to a deeper knowledge about the interaction between the forces behind an observed pattern. This may only be analyzed through intensive and focused studies of deliberately selected cases. Any quest for certitude or "fixed correlations" between social variables must be jettisoned (Bhaskar, 1998).

Retroduction, a research strategy used by critical realists, is more like a thought experiment than an inference. It is an inference form, based on a given event, that reflects on necessary conditions and deep causal relations that must exist before the event occurred. In this reflection process, it is necessary to divide the relevant from the contingent. What must exist for this to happen?

Emergent properties at different levels of reality

Social work practices often search for interconnectedness between the personal and the social, between biography and history. We use the concept of a laminated system to ontologically underpin a critique of the history of micro-social studies involving three successive forms of reductionism: medical reductionism, psychological reductionism, and cultural reductionism. Bhaskar and Danermark's contribution in this book (Chapter 4) argues for the concept of "*a necessarily laminated system*" to emphasize that some levels cannot be excluded in the analysis without committing to the fallacy of reductionism.

In philosophy, systems theory, science, and art, *emergence* is conceived as a situation or a process whereby larger entities, patterns, and regularities arise through interactions among smaller or simpler entities that themselves do not exhibit such properties. A family's interaction is a result of each member's actions and interaction in the system. If a member changes his or her behavior, the interaction pattern in the family also changes.

Emergence is the process whereby the global behavior of a system results from the actions and interactions of agents. There are *emergent properties* at each level of reality, where new properties and causal powers develop (by emergence) at each level, compared with the level below. The causal powers from the lower levels also exist in the higher levels. The different levels often make up research areas for each different discipline. How one divides into different levels depends on the research topic. The division into different levels is a social construction and belongs to the transitive dimension of the reality. However, the phenomenon emerges that new causal powers develop depending on whether the levels below belong to the intransitive dimension of the reality. Examples could include traffic jams, the V-shape of bird flocks, and colonies of social insects (Sawyer, 2009).

The basic ideal for mechanist explanations must be to picture the causal chain or process that explains how a particular social phenomenon was brought about. However, the concept of causal chain does not imply a linear view of causal processes. The causal process can be a constellation of individuals and their actions and interactions (for instance, a network) that brings forth a particular social structure. Otherwise, individuals are influenced by society through socialization in the first phase and affect the same society through their interactions in the next phase. In our opinion, this is exactly what characterizes generative mechanisms. However, we are usually unable to observe these mechanisms in detail; we then need plausible theories of the middle range to explain the relationship.

Studying social emergence means exploring the emergence processes of the micro-macro link. Professionals in counseling work are interested in processes because they focus on change over time. The unit of analysis is *situated practice*, rather than the bounded individual, and focus on practice includes both the person and the structural and cultural factors. The individual and the group cannot be studied in isolation, but only in situated practice where they are embedded. Sawyer (2009) argued that societies are complex dynamical systems and that the best way to resolve these debates is by developing the concept of emergence, paying attention to multiple levels of analysis – individuals, interactions, and groups – with a dynamic focus on how social group phenomena emerge from communication processes among individual members. Social emergence is the link between interaction with stable and ephemeral emergence. A focus on social emergence requires an interdisciplinary approach when analyzing both individuals and collectives. One example is a boy who has been diagnosed with attention deficit/hyperactivity disorder (ADHD). His problems have both biological (neuropsychological) and cognitive (psychological) causes. The schoolteachers and pupils see him as a difficult boy who does not listen. We may see that he is trapped in an interactive category as being "difficult", so it is important to be aware of what categorizations do to individuals who become trapped in them. He has problems understanding messages; therefore, conflicts emerge in his milieu. His problems may now be seen as interactional problems, viewing them from a broad, relational perspective that incorporates biological, psychological, social, and material insights into the problems.

References

Archer, M. S. (2000) *Being Human: The Problem of Agency*, Cambridge: Cambridge University Press.

Archer, M. S. (2003) *Structure, Agency and the Internal Conversation*, Cambridge: Cambridge University Press.

Archer, M. S., Bhaskar, R., Collier, A., Lawson, T., Norrie, A., Bhaskar, R., Collier, A., Lawson, T., & Norrie, A. (1998) *Critical Realism: Essential Readings*, London: Routledge

Bhaskar, R. (1978) *A Realist Theory of Science*, Brighton: Harvester Press.

Bhaskar, R. (1986) *Scientific Realism & Human Emancipation*, London: Verso.

Bhaskar, R. (1998) *The Possibility of Naturalism*, London: Routledge.

Brian-Lawson, K. (2012) Response: Critical realism: Response to Longhofer and Floersch, *Research on Social Work Practice*, 22(5), 523–528, doi:10.1177/1049731512454015.

Buch-Hansen, H., & Nielsen, P. (2005) *Kritisk Realisme* [Critical Realism], Frederiksberg: Roskilde Universitetsforlag.

Danermark, B., Ekström, M., Jakobsen, L., & Karlsson, J. C. (2002) *Explaining Society: Critical Realism in the Social Sciences*, London: Routledge.

Fleetwood, S. (2004) An Ontology for Organization and Management Studies. In Fleetwood, S. & Ackroyd, S. (eds.), *The Ontology of Organisational and Management Studies*, London: Routledge.

Houston, S. (2001) Transcending the fissure in risk theory: Critical realism and child welfare, *Child and Family Social Work*, 6, 219–228.

Houston, S. (2012) Response: Reviewing the coming crisis in social work: A response to Longhofer and Floersch, *Research on Social Work Practice*, 22(5), 520–522, doi:10.1177/1049731512441264.

Kalleberg, R. (1992) *A Constructive Turn in Sociology*, Oslo: Department of Sociology, University of Oslo.

Krauss, S. E. (2005) Research paradigms and meaning making: A primer, *The Qualitative Report*, 4, 758–770.

Morén, S., & Blom, B. (2003) Explaining human change: On generative mechanisms in social work practice, *Journal of Critical Realism*, 2(1), 37–60.

Sawyer, K. (2009) *Social Emergence: Societies as Complex Systems*, Cambridge: Cambridge University Press.

Sayer, A. (1992) *Method in Social Science: A Realist Approach*, London: Routledge.

Sayer, A. (2000; 2008) *Realism and Social Science*, London: Sage.

Part II

3 Normativity in the social sciences and professions[1]

Andrew Sayer

Introduction

In everyday life, the most important questions we face tend to be normative ones about what is good or bad, right or wrong. Because of our psychological and physical vulnerability, our dependence on others, and our capacity for diverse actions, our relation to the world is one of concern, for we can flourish or suffer. We are necessarily *evaluative beings*, continually having to monitor and evaluate how we, and other things we care about, are faring, often wondering 'what to do for the best', whether it is about our health, our actions, our environment or our relations with others. Some of this evaluation is done 'on automatic', semi-consciously, in the flow of life, but some involves reflection or 'internal conversations' (Archer, 2003). Evaluation is central to the work of professionals such as social workers, who continually assess the well-being and safety or otherwise of clients, and decide what they need and what would improve their situation.

However, in social science, positive (descriptive and explanatory) questions are primary, and indeed normative judgements are widely seen as radically different, and in danger of compromising the objectivity of research. The orthodox position is that facts and value are sharply distinct, values cannot be derived from facts, and it is not the job of social science to make value judgements. In addition, even though social science generally recognizes that values and valuation pervade the worlds of those they study, its treatment of people's relation to the world of concern often fails to do justice to it. Typically, it either reduces their behaviour to the following of conventions or norms, or treats values as merely subjective, and not about anything objective. People's values and evaluations are seen as just facts about them, not beliefs and claims that have import or significance and could be more or less true. The result is an alienated and alienating representation of social life that fails to acknowledge the force of people's concerns and evaluations. Moreover, if a social scientific account of a situation fails to tell us whether people are flourishing or suffering – because its authors believe they must not make value judgements in their work – the account will inevitably be deficient as a description.

The inadequacy of these treatments of normativity is evident in many everyday situations. When a social worker says a child is being abused, this clearly involves not only an evaluative judgement that the situation is *bad* but also a factual claim about what is the case; she is not merely arbitrarily projecting a value judgement onto the world or just following a convention or norm. It straddles any distinction of fact and value. And on the basis of what she believes to be fact, the social worker has to decide what action should be taken; she appears to derive an *ought* from an *is*. And of course in life generally, we continually have to make judgements about situations and decide what to do.

In this chapter, I shall argue that if social science is to understand both everyday life and the work of professionals, it needs to overcome its resistance to normativity, both as part of its object of study and within its own practice or discourse. If it is to understand people and their world, it needs to take the normative dimension of life seriously, both in terms of how and why things matter to people, and recognize that evaluative judgements may be more or less true. This involves challenging the pervasive assumption that positive and normative thought, or fact and value, are always radically distinct and incompatible. While it involves some arguments from critical realism, the argument also draws upon literature from neo-Aristotelian ethics and the ethic of care. I shall first argue that social science's dominant understanding of the nature of values is flawed, and that its dichotomous treatments of fact and value are unsustainable where issues of health or flourishing or suffering concerned. I shall then discuss whether some valuations – for example, about well-being – might have universal applicability or whether all such judgements are culturally specific. Next, I argue that acting ethically requires attentiveness to the specificities of the other and their context, and go on to illustrate this in relation to care and dignity. Penultimately, I discuss and critique poststructuralism's own difficulties with normativity, before concluding.

Social science and values

In so far as social science deals with normativity, it tends to treat people's sentiments, concerns and judgements just as contingent facts about them and their societies. Their values are either just subjective, individual preferences ('emotivism')[2] or internalised social norms ('conventionalism'). In neither case are they seen as rational or as responses to objective states of affairs, such as practices of kindness or cruelty. In conventionalism, values are merely arbitrary cultural conventions – 'what people do round here' – or in a more recent version, merely 'culturally constituted'. As Davydova and Sharrock note, this 'implies a 'conformity concept of morality' (Davydova & Sharrock, 2003; see also Bauman, 1989). Consequently, it can render people as socially constructed dupes – objects of a superior sociological gaze. In both emotivist and conventionalist interpretations, the normative force of individuals' concerns and valuations – how and why they matter to actors – is lost, edited out, as if it were either unimportant or too obvious to require comment.

However, both approaches seem at least half-right. Values are subjective in the sense that they are important elements of individuals' characters and beliefs; they may be shared with others, but they are also felt personally. In addition, conventionalism acknowledges that values vary significantly across societies, and that individuals tend to take on the values of their own culture. Yet, while values are indeed culturally variable, they are not completely arbitrary; they have something to do with well-being and ill-being and they refer to something which is not merely their product. When those who are subjectivists or conventionalists in the seminar room experience bad treatment by someone in their everyday lives, they are unlikely to remonstrate with the perpetrator by saying, 'Look, personally, I just don't happen to like that', or 'Don't you know that's culturally constructed as bad round here?'; rather they are likely to draw attention in some way to the harm and suffering that has been caused. This implies that values are not just conventions about what we should do and think but about matters to do with well-being, where well-being is not simply anything we care to define it as or just an experience, but a state which can exist even if it is not noticed, and which we can try to understand, or construct if it has not been achieved. To refer to harm is to identify objective consequences. To be sure, our sensitivity to and awareness of harm is mediated by available ways of seeing and convention, and our beliefs about harm are fallible, but that fallibility presupposes there is something objective in the sense of independent of our beliefs about which we can be mistaken (Collier, 2003). At the same time, if we could never successfully identify harm, we wouldn't survive for long. We tell our children to be careful when crossing the road not because in our culture it is constructed as dangerous, but because it is dangerous whatever our culture, and the costs of our fallibility in making judgements about it are extremely high.

In other words, our values and value judgements, particularly those concerning how people relate to one another, have a *eudaimonistic* content, to use Aristotle's term: that is, they involve an assessment of flourishing or its absence. Many social norms are based upon beliefs about what constitutes human flourishing, though some appear to be no more than arbitrary conventions. As Shaun Nichols shows, research on how people make ethical judgements shows them to be capable of distinguishing eudaimonistic moral norms or values from conventional or authority-based norms. He reports an interesting study by Nucci of Amish children in the United States in which it was found that 100% of them 'said that if God had made no rule against working on Sunday, it would not be wrong to work on Sunday. However, more than 80% of these subjects said that even if God had made no rule about hitting, it would still be wrong to hit' (Nichols, 2004, p. 6). Other studies of children have shown them to be able to distinguish the moral from the merely conventional by their third birthday (Nichols, 2004, p. 78). Interestingly, studies of psychopaths have shown them to be incapable of distinguishing the moral from the conventional, since they think of all wrongdoing in terms of the transgression of norms. By contrast, non-psychopathic criminals are able to appreciate that their actions were wrong not merely because they transgressed norms or conventions but because they harmed others (Nichols, 2004, p. 76). How interesting too that some sociologists should support the idea that actions are only wrong because they are socially defined as wrong![3] Sociologists may sometimes cite actors' moral terms in inverted commas to indicate that they are not endorsing the judgements those terms imply, but it is a mistake to allow this methodological device to become an ontological assumption that they are just conventions rather than judgements about suffering or well-being (Davydova & Sharrock, 2003).

To understand normativity in life we need a conception of people which sees them as capable but vulnerable sentient beings, having needs and wants that are in continual need of replenishment or development. We are always poised between existing mixes of lack, suffering and flourishing and possible future ones, and always in varying degrees aware of our situation and concerned about it. This implies what might, for want of a better term, be called a 'needs-based conception of social being' and action, viewing actors not only as causal agents and as self-interpreting meaning makers but as needy, desiring beings, dependent on others, having an orientation to the world of care and concern[4] and capable of flourishing or suffering. 'Needs' here is used as a shorthand that also covers lack, wants and desire.[5] While some have mainly physiological origins, others might be termed 'culturally-acquired or emergent needs' deriving from involvement in and commitment to cultural practices, such as the need of the religious to worship.

There are some common sources of reluctance to embrace such a conception. One is the fear – often driven by sociological imperialism – that acknowledging needs, drives and the like implies essentialism, biologism and psychologism.[6] Yet a reference to needs and the like does not have to imply that they are reducible to inborn bodily or psychological requirements, for although we are born with some basic needs, even these are quickly socially cultivated and developed, and culturally interpreted and mediated. Contrary to a common misconception in much philosophy and social science, including post-structuralism, nature is not immutable. Consequently, to acknowledge that we have biological causal powers and liabilities is not to submit to biological determinism, for as with any living being, our interactions with our environment can modify as well as reproduce those powers. In particular, neuroplasticity means that our brains are continually being reshaped by our experiences, though at any moment, just how they are affected by them depends on what our brains currently allow. So we can reject a cultural determinism that treats people's characteristics as having nothing to do with their biology. Needs, lack and vulnerability presuppose not determinism but the *openness* of the world, for there is always the possibility of *failure* to satisfy, fulfil or endure. In critical realist terms, we live in open systems, whose future is not predetermined. Moreover, although lack is inescapable, we can to some extent shape what form our needs and desires take, though wishful thinking has limits. Nor does acknowledging biological powers and liabilities entail a homogenisation of human needs and wants, for each of us is different and we are capable of a vast range of forms of life. Furthermore, as we noted, many needs and wants are effectively culturally autonomous and irreducible, though these too presuppose a capacity for acculturation not possessed by many other species.

The treatment of meaning within the needs-based approach goes beyond that of hermeneutic approaches in that it deals with not only signifiers and the signified, and shared understandings, but *significance* or *import*. This is what people refer to when they talk about 'what something means to them', such as what their friends mean to them or what it means to be an immigrant (Sayer, 2006). In such cases, they are not giving a definition of those things, but an indication of their import or significance for them, how they value them, how such things impact on their well-being or something else that they care about (Taylor, 1985). The relationship to the world that is implied is one of care or concern and valuation, in which things are assessed for their implications for well-being, however defined. Here, emotions, understood not only as 'affect' but as embodied commentaries on our well-being and concerns, are fundamental to understanding what makes us care about and want to do anything, and what makes anything matter (Archer, 2000; Nussbaum, 2001). An ethnographic study might explain, in a matter-of-fact way, how the members of a certain group understand and act toward each other in terms of meanings primarily as conventions or shared interpretations, but give little indication of just why some things have particular import or significance for them, that is how they affect things they care about.[7]

'What something means to me' cannot reasonably be glossed merely as subjective; the evaluations and feelings are *about* something, including the well-being or ill-being of actors, and perhaps the fortunes of particular practices and institutions. We also assume that those subjective beliefs and feelings that we and others have are objective in the sense that they do exist. While they tell us something about the valuer, they are justified (or not) by reference to claims about the nature of their objects, and thus are descriptive as well as evaluative. Any account of social practices which gives no indication of their implications for well-being, if only in terms of correcting a misapprehension, invites responses like 'so what?', 'what's your point?' The editing out of significance, perhaps because it is felt to be 'unscientific', is a central cause of the alienated character of so much contemporary social science.

Beyond the fact-value dichotomy

Social science's difficulties in understanding the normative dimension of social life derive from the influence of certain philosophical ideas about facts and values. These include: 1) that facts and values are radically distinct such that while factual claims can be true or false, value judgements about what is good or bad cannot; and 2) that value judgements about what is good or bad or what we ought to do, cannot be derived from facts. Although these ideas are actually contested in philosophy (e.g. Putnam, 2002; Taylor, 1973; Williams, 1985), few social scientists realise this, and so they are allowed an extraordinary privilege.

Under the influence of these claims, social scientists are traditionally taught to distinguish sharply between fact and value; the belief that this can and must be done tends to become deeply engrained. While researchers can study values, they are generally taught that they must try to minimise the effect of their own values in their accounts, and to abstain from value judgements, so that they can be objective. Radicals tend to oppose this by inverting it: they say that no one can be value-free, so they won't pretend to be objective. Yet, of course, they don't just make up their research results and they clearly believe their accounts to be truer than those they reject. The problem here is that both conservatives and their radical opponents agree that objectivity and value judgements cannot go together.

We can begin to see what is wrong with this assumption by going back to the example of the social worker's claim that 'this child is being abused'. This is a truth claim – a fallible claim about a state of affairs that is objective in the sense of capable of existing regardless of whether it is observed or understood by anyone. Indeed, as critical realists argue, it is precisely because of this independence of many states of affairs from their being observed by someone that makes knowledge of them fallible (Collier, 2003). The claim is based on a judgement, and in that sense is 'subjective', but this doesn't mean it cannot be more or less 'objective' in the different sense of 'true'. The social worker obviously has values and is aware of certain norms about how children should be treated. However, those norms aren't merely arbitrary conventions; they are based on judgements about flourishing and suffering, and what is good or bad for children. So is the social worker's claim a factual one or a value judgement, or both?

When we talk about people and their actions, we often use words which seem to combine fact and value, description and evaluation; we describe them as kind, cruel, courageous, generous, selfish, humiliating, racist, abusive, oppressive and so on. These are 'thick ethical descriptions'. If you don't know that humiliation or cruelty are *bad,* you don't know what they *are*; the descriptive and evaluative components can't be separated. Thus, when we decide to accept a description of some practice, say, as 'abusive' or 'racist', we simultaneously accept the implicit valuation. By comparison, *thin* ethical concepts such as 'good,',' bad', 'duty', 'virtue', 'obligation', 'right' and 'wrong' ('empty moral words', as Iris Murdoch called them) can seem more like arbitrary assertions than reasonable descriptions and evaluations (Murdoch, 1970, p. 40). This is precisely because as abstractions and summarising terms, thin ethical terms are removed from the range of concrete situations and behaviours to which they might be applied and in terms of which they can be justified (Putnam, 2002, p. 60). In addition, it is this abstraction from concrete aspects of life which lends credence to the idea that all evaluative claims are radically distinct from factual claims. Yet, where issues of well-being are concerned, we encounter a middle ground between fact and value.

Part of the problem is a common misunderstanding of 'values' that reduces them to purely subjective phenomena, ignoring the fact that they are *about* things that can exist largely independently of them. It is clearer in the case of 'valuation' and 'evaluation' that these have objects, or referents. It is easier to overlook the referents of values than those of specific evaluations, because values are more abstract – they are sedimented valuations that have become attitudes or dispositions, and which recursively inform particular evaluations or judgements we make on specific occasions. Sometimes we are scarcely aware of some of our values, but they influence particular evaluations that we make of events. Although our values tend to be deeply embrained or embodied, they can be changed. For example, it is possible for our negative values about a certain kind of person to be challenged if they behave in ways that we did not expect of them, generating cognitive dissonance. Particularly if the experience is repeated, our values may change, though habits of thought can take a long time to revise. Hence, though they are often difficult to argue about, values are not beyond reason. Typically, when we reason about them we do so by reference to the actions and circumstances to which they refer, for example, by pointing to problems that are produced by a certain kind of behaviour, such as those associated with drug dependency.

When we turn to the idea that values cannot be derived from facts, usually referred to as the 'is/ought problem', we immediately notice that this middle ground is missing: evaluation – which spans both description and evaluation – is ignored and normativity is reduced to imperative direction – 'should', 'ought'. It is then argued that values cannot be logically derived from facts, and that social scientists should not attempt to derive any normative conclusions from empirical research. For example, from the fact that, someone has no home, it doesn't logically (i.e. deductively) follow that they should have one. However, deductive logic is highly demanding and in not only everyday life but in science we make inferences that are not arrived at through deduction. Indeed, it is bizarre to insist on such a demanding criterion for inferring what to do. Imagine going to the doctor to have your blood pressure taken. She does so and gives you two numbers, one over the other. You say, 'is that good or bad? What should I do about it?' Imagine if the doctor answered, 'Well, I can't tell you because that would be a value judgement and it would compromise my objectivity, and I can't advise you what to do because you can't derive an ought from an is.'

This shows the absurdity of dichotomising fact and value in such cases, and of assuming that the only inferences that we can rely on are deductive ones. The fact that ought does not follow deductively from is, is purely of academic interest. Logic is about the relation between statements, not about the causal relations between things like your blood pressure and your well-being. Similarly, if you are hungry, you need food, not because of any logical relationship between statements about these things, but because your body lacks food and is telling you to get some. 'The force of the ought' here comes from the causal processes. We could not survive, let alone flourish, if we did not regularly derive conclusions about what is good and bad, and what we should do, from our observations of states of affairs. Those judgements are fallible, of course, but then so too are simple factual claims.

Values and universalism

As I noted earlier, conventionalist views of values are common in social science because it is particularly clear in such research that values vary significantly between different societies, and that different ways of life are associated with different value systems and define well-being in different ways. Such a realisation does not fit easily with claims that we can resolve value disputes by reference to a common set of characteristics constituting human well-being, for this might be taken to presuppose a common, universal human nature and to ignore cultural variation. On the other hand, it has to be accepted that, as Mary Midgley says, 'you can't have a plant or an animal without certain quite definite things being good and bad for it' (Midgley, 2003, p. 54), and in everyday life it's important to be able to distinguish among these with some degree of success just to survive. Yet some may still object that we don't know what well-being is, for we are always judging this from a limited perspective in human culture and history.

We need to steer a course between a universalism that ignores cultural difference and a conventionalism that implies that the collective wishful thinking of any culture can make any practice good and enable flourishing. The first step is to recognize that our remarkable capacity for cultural variation implies that we have something in common, which things like insects or rocks don't have. For example, regardless of where it was born, a baby can be taught any of the world's thousands of languages; a child born to English parents in London that was immediately given to Japanese parents in Tokyo would learn Japanese as easily as Japanese-born children do. Therefore, babies must have *similar* capacities to be able to become so *different*. To be sure, children vary in their linguistic abilities, just as in their physiques, but they have important similarities without which acculturation could not be explained. Furthermore, the fact that particular cultural practices have similar effects on groups of people exposed to them suggests the latter share similar capacities and susceptibilities.

The second step is to acknowledge that we have 'differently-cultivated natures', which have adjusted to particular ways of life that produce certain common patterns of wants and needs, and corresponding sources of flourishing and suffering. Thus, someone deeply religious may be harmed if they are prevented from praying, whereas for an atheist, compulsory religious observance is a form of oppression. Different cultures provide both different ways of life and different interpretations of life and what is good or bad. But while they may enable different kinds of flourishing, not just any cultural practice enables well-being: some things like foot-binding or child abuse or eating junk food cause damage regardless of whether a particular culture believes them to be good. And given the fallibility of our present knowledge and the possibility of new forms of society, there may be forms of well-being that we have yet to discover. However, this doesn't mean we know *nothing* about human well-being – we must beware of the all-or-nothing fallacy, that unless we know everything about something, we know nothing. We know that we need food and shelter, that children need love and security to be able to become confident social actors, that workers need time for their bodies to recover, that freedom from the threat of violence is important for well-being, that a degree of autonomy is important for human dignity, and so on. It would be fatuous to deny such things.

In other words, in accordance with the capability approach, there are certain things (capabilities) – beings and doings – that we must have the freedom to do if we are to flourish (Sen, 1999; Nussbaum, 2000). The way in which these capabilities are understood and provided may differ between cultures, but they have something in common. Thus, the need for recognition and respect can be met in different ways in different cultures, according to their particular traditions. This, then, is a pluralist and objectivist view, in keeping with critical realism, but not a relativist one. It argues that there are many forms of well-being, but not that well-being simply depends on one's cultural point of view.

Attending to the specificities of the other

As we have seen, critical realism sees values as being about something that can exist independently of them, and as capable of being more or less true or appropriate for those states of affairs. In this respect, it has similarities to both Aristotelianism, which holds that, notwithstanding cultural difference, humans have some capacities for flourishing and suffering in common. And both of these approaches share with the feminist ethic of care a conception of good ethical behaviour that involves attending to the specificities of the other and the context, rather than simply following rules or norms to the letter regardless of the details of a particular case (Kittay, 1999; Tronto, 1994). For these three approaches, rules are at best 'guidelines' that may work in many common situations, but have to be adjusted appropriately to take account of differences. Andrew Collier, a critical realist, argues that the role of rules in ethics is limited to obvious things such as prohibitions on torture and murder:

> The main body of ethics cannot be formulated in such rules, but will consist in recognising the complexity and specificity of every human being . . . . Moral codes which consist of do-s and don't-s serve mainly to excuse their adherents from thinking about how they should treat this particular being in this particular situation.
>
> (Collier, 1999, p. 91)

Good carers or social workers, like skilled surgeons, are distinguished by their ability to deal sensitively with difference. Rules and prescribed procedures may be helpful to novices for beginning to learn how to be a nurse, social worker or surgeon, but they soon learn more through practice than by following rules. Experts tend not to follow them, and indeed doing so might impede them and result in less efficient and poorer quality work. Although it's also possible for experienced practitioners to become complacent and make mistakes, the tendency of management of professionals to respond by making them follow formal procedures to the letter can be counterproductive.

Paradoxically, in this view, critical realists like Collier (1999) and Sayer (2011)[8] argue that 'norms' should *not* be seen as the essence of normativity, though in some social practices they may be given absolute status. At best, they codify common moral responses that have been tried out and validated publicly as forms of wisdom. However, as Collier says, precisely because slavish norm following can become a substitute for attending to the situation at hand, this is risky.

Care and dignity

Attending ethically to the specificities of the other involves protecting their dignity. This matters hugely to people. Though they may take it for granted if their dignity is respected, if it is not, they are likely to be deeply troubled. Dignity is commonly invoked both in declarations of human rights and by oppressed groups appealing for support, but it is rarely defined. Recently, though, certain professional bodies have become more aware of its importance, for their work involves intervention in others' lives in the context of a power-differential between practitioner and client. Unless this is handled sensitively, it can undermine clients' dignity. Consequently, there have recently been attempts to specify what dignity involves in the spheres of life they represent.[9]

Most commonly, dignity is associated with the idea of individuals having autonomy in the sense of self-command, and hence as having their own goals or ends that need to be respected by others. Our dignity is denied us if others use us wholly as means to their ends. And we cannot have dignity if no one listens to us and takes what we say seriously. To have dignity we must be allowed to act according to our own will and reasoning, provided we take due consideration of others' dignity. However, as the latter qualification implies, this autonomy is not unlimited or reducible to simple independence. We are social beings, in varying degrees and ways dependent on each other. To respect someone's dignity is also to trust them to use their autonomy in a way that takes account of others, and their dignity. It includes trusting them to take on responsibilities competently and in good faith. Those who are not trusted or act in ways which betray trust lack dignity.

Dignity is also commonly associated with competence – with having capacities and being able to act effectively. However, this implies that our dignity is threatened if we lose some of the capacities that we once had, particularly if they are normally associated with flourishing. For example, someone who has lost their hearing or become incontinent may feel their dignity is threatened, especially if others fail to take appropriate account of this change or take advantage of their vulnerability. Dignity is therefore not only about autonomy and capacities but vulnerabilities. Good care is sensitive to both capacities and vulnerabilities, and treats the patient in ways that gives recognition to the former without drawing undue attention to the latter.

Above all, respecting and supporting someone's dignity involves recognizing them as a whole person, with a history, achievements, needs, concerns, commitments and relationships to others that matter to them, and being attentive to their words and feelings. Care or other work with people that disregards this and reduces clients to a set of characteristics that a professional unilaterally decides need to be dealt with undermines their dignity.

While it is common, particularly in liberal societies to talk of dignity as a given quality of individuals, these considerations show that it is relational – dependent on interactions with others. As such, it is fragile: it is a basic need whose fulfilment depends on the kind of relationships people have to others, may or may not be realised, rather than something that is simply already realised in everyone regardless of this.

Post-structuralism's misunderstandings of normativity

Much of the above is at odds with the understandings of values, normativity and human social being that are dominant in social science in the tradition of Foucault. While he was renowned for being a tireless political activist, campaigning against various forms of oppression, as an academic Foucault refused to evaluate the practices he studied, and his writings are notably devoid of thick ethical concepts. Although he compellingly demonstrated how power or power/knowledge constructs as well as constrains, and can produce pleasure, he refused to distinguish between benign and harmful forms of construction or constraint: democracy therefore appears no better than dictatorship. His accounts generally have an ominous tone, yet they fail to indicate what, if anything, is problematic in the practices he studied. Hence, some authors have criticized his work for being 'crypto-normative' (Fraser, 1989; Habermas, 1990). But it is also crypto-descriptive, for if an account of social life doesn't at least implicitly indicate whether there is flourishing or suffering and injustice, it doesn't tell us very much. Not surprisingly he was often questioned about this. As he stated on one occasion:

> The role of an intellectual is not to tell others what they have to do. By what right would he do so? The work of the intellectual is not to shape others' political will: it is, through the analyses that he carried out in his own field, to question over and over again what is postulated as self-evident, to disturb people's mental habits, the way they do and think things.
>
> (Foucault, 1997, p. 131)

It is clear from this and from elsewhere that Foucault (mis)understood normativity as a matter of 'oughts'; like positivists arguing about values in social science via the is-ought relation, he reduced normativity to imperatives and ignored the more important and prior part – evaluation.

In post-structuralism, including queer theory, normativity is associated with *normalising*, particularly because the latter imposes identity categories that have the effect of suppressing difference, for example, marginalizing and stigmatising inter-sex people. But instead of resisting the prior reduction of normativity to norms, or challenging just those forms of normalising that have unfair effects, normativity in general is condemned on this ground and rejected. Yet, of course, this is contradictory for being against normativity is itself a normative stance. Life is normative in the sense of continually requiring evaluation and judgements about how to act. It's inescapable. To be against sexism, homophobia and racism is to be normative. And some 'abnormal' behaviours, such as child abuse, are indeed harmful: not all differences are good, and hence not all normalising is problematic. Regardless of whether behaviours are normal or abnormal in the sense of common or uncommon, we have to assess them in terms of their implications for justice and well-being. But then, as we have argued, norms should not be the heart of ethics: again, we need to attend to the other, their needs, susceptibilities and capacities, and their situation.

However, there are deeper obstacles to understanding normativity in post-structuralism, which lie in its social ontology and its non-realist tendencies. In reacting against the straw 'humanist' figure of the individual as an independent, sovereign, coherent, unified agent responding to an external world as it freely chooses, post-structuralism gives us a demeaning view of 'subjects' as wholly the product of social forces – not just constrained and enabled by them but constituted by them. Even where subjects engage in 'care of the self', they do so in ways which overwhelmingly involve conforming with wider 'force-relations', discourse or 'power/knowledge'.

In part, this is right: we are indeed constituted through our interactions with the wider world, from the moment of conception to our deaths. And post-structuralism has usefully drawn attention to the importance of the 'micro-physics' of power in everyday life in shaping who we are and what we do. But at every moment, our susceptibility to these interactions or forces depends on the powers of our mind-bodies, as these have so far co-evolved. And these powers go beyond physiological and psychological limits to include *reflexivity* – the ability to consider ourselves in relation to our social contexts, and vice versa (Archer, 2007). We do not have to flip from the caricature of the sovereign reasoner to the cultural dope, whether the latter appears in traditional sociological guise or in post-structuralist form. We do not simply submit equally to any kind of treatment, regardless of its relation to us or what we think about it: some influences may get below our radar, but others can be resisted, welcomed or redirected according to how they fit with our bodies and our dispositions, beliefs, commitments and concerns.

Morality and ethics are not reducible to internalized conventions or norms, and they can challenge the latter. As Michael Walzer explains:

> The moral world and the social world are more or less coherent, but they are never more than more or less coherent. Morality is always potentially subversive of class and power.
>
> (Walzer, 1989, p. 22)

Our moral sentiments are not just products of prevailing forms of power, but are the co-products of our mind-bodies, our physiology – for example, the mirror neurons which enable empathy – and our capacities to feel and think, as these have been influenced by, and have engaged with, our culture. All of these are co-products of social, biological and physical interactions. As Kate Soper comments:

> [T]he body is neither simply the effect of discourse nor simply a point of 'brute' resistance to it, but a centre of experience which is actively involved in the construction of discourse itself. . . . Instinct and feeling, both physical and emotional, everywhere intrude to influence what is said – just as the things which come to be said intrude back upon feeling.
>
> (Soper, 1990, p. 11)

It is one thing to reject the idea that we are sovereign individual subjects, guided by reason, coherent and internally unified, somehow already constituted prior to socialization; it is quite another to reduce people to ciphers, faceless 'subjects' or 'bodies', objects of a superior yet curiously unreflexive academic gaze.

Finally, post-structuralism's difficulties with normativity are underpinned by its overly strong form of social constructionism which assumes that discourses produce what they name, unilaterally and successfully, as if collective wishful thinking – 'regimes of truth' – always worked. However, while discourses can sometimes do this to some degree, there are invariably resistances, intractable objects and unintended consequences, and simply many other things going on. Thus, a child who is taken into care by social workers may come to understand herself in the terms used by social workers and adopt an identity in foster care as a 'looked after child' (in the UK), and this may influence her behaviour, yet this does not simply replace the many other aspects of her identity and ways of thinking about them but exists in tension with them (Denenberg, 2016). Discourses as ways of thinking embedded and enacted in practices and institutions produce real effects, but like any knowledge, discourses are fallible; as critical realism insists, the world is not reducible to our knowledge of it, nor does it submit to our interventions if these do not fit with its powers.

Conclusion

I have been proposing a view of normativity not in terms of norms and imperatives or free-floating values but as an ongoing process in the flow of life through which we monitor and evaluate things in relation to needs, wants, commitments and concerns, or more generally in relation to well-being. The verbal expression of these evaluations usually involves thick ethical concepts that defy any fact-value dichotomy. However, this dichotomy is deeply ingrained in modernity, as part of a family of such hierarchical oppositions: objective/subjective, mind/body, reason/emotion, science/ethics. Thus, emotions are seen not as intelligent responses to the world but as irrational and unreasonable. In social science, there has been an attempt to expel values from science and reason, and while there have been radical challenges to this, these often leave the dichotomy intact as we saw. What is less noticed is the attempted expulsion of reason from values, and it is this in particular that we need to challenge. One important reason why social science is poor at recognizing this is that the dichotomies have become an organizing principle of the division of academic knowledge as it has developed over the last 150 years, so that normative thinking has become ghettoized in philosophy and political theory, while the other disciplines assume that they can and should disregard it (Sayer, 2000b). The work of professionals like social workers is inescapably normative, but so too is life in general. Directly or indirectly, our evaluative judgements are related to well-being, including matters of fairness and justice. In turn, well-being is constrained and enabled by our differently cultivated natures, by the kind of beings we have become. Whether to understand society, or to intervene in it as professionals, or just to live well, we need to study and evaluate these matters.

Notes

1 This chapter draws extensively on my book *Why Things Matter to People* (Sayer, 2011).
2 'Emotivism is the doctrine that all evaluative judgments and more specifically all moral judgments are nothing but expressions of preference, expressions of attitude or feeling, insofar as they are moral or evaluative in character . . . [they] are neither true nor false; and agreement in moral judgment is not to be secured by any rational method, for there are none. . . . We use moral judgments not only to express our own feelings or attitudes, but also precisely to produce such effects in others' (MacIntyre, 1985, pp. 11–12). As we shall see, the term is unfortunate in that it suggests emotions have nothing to do with reason.
3 This subjectivist view of values goes back 2,300 years to Epicurus, and is reproduced in Durkheim's claim that 'actions are evil because they are socially prohibited, rather than socially prohibited because they are evil' (Bauman, 1989, p. 173).
4 There are some similarities here with Heidegger's emphasis on care in *Being and Time* (Heidegger, 1962).
5 Needs, lack and desire cannot be assimilated comfortably just to critical realism's concepts of causal powers and liabilities, for these are not simply powers to do or suffer change: rather they imply impulses or drives to remove the deficiencies they represent. Although following Bhaskar's later work, some critical realists may want to use the concept of 'absence' here (Bhaskar, 1993), in my view, this effectively invents a concept (in non-realist fashion) as a substitute for identifying the mechanisms that produce and satisfy needs.
6 On essentialism and anti-essentialism, see O'Neill (1994) and Sayer (2000a).
7 Renato Rosaldo has noted this tendency in anthropology (Rosaldo, 1989).
8 Critical realists are not unique in demoting norms in ethics (e.g. Dancy, 2004), and one prominent critical realist – Dave Elder-Vass – gives norms considerable prominence (Elder-Vass, 2012).
9 Social Care Institute for Excellence, 2013; Shotton & Seedhouse, 1998. Trade unions have also begun to put dignity on their agendas and to define what it means. See, for example, Unison trade union's Dignity at Work campaign in the UK, and The Workplace Dignity Institute in South Africa. See Unite the Union (2014) Zero Tolerance: Dignity at Work, www.unitetheunion.org/uploaded/documents/ZeroToleranceGuide11-18154.pdf

References

Archer, M.S. (2000) *Being Human,* Cambridge: Cambridge University Press.
Archer, M. S. (2003) *Structure, Agency and the Internal Conversation*, Cambridge: Cambridge University Press.
Archer, M. S. (2007) *Making Our Way Through the World*, Cambridge: Cambridge University Press.
Bauman, Z. (1989) *Modernity and the Holocaust*, Cambridge: Polity Press.
Bhaskar, R. (1993) *Dialectic: The Pulse of Freedom*, London: Verso.
Collier, A. (1999) *Being and Worth*, London: Routledge.
Collier, A. (2003) *In Defence of Objectivity*, London: Routledge.
Dancy, J. (2004) *Ethics Without Principles*, Oxford: Oxford University Press.
Davydova, I., & Sharrock, W. (2003) The rise and fall of the fact/value distinction, *The Sociological Review*, 51(3), 357–375.
Denenberg, P. (2016) The Experience of Children and Young People in Long Term Foster Care, Ph.D. Thesis, Lancaster University.
Elder-Vass, D. (2012) *The Reality of Social Construction*, Cambridge: Cambridge University Press.

Foucault, M. (1997) What Is Critique? In Lotringer, S. & Hochroth, L. (eds.), *The Politics of Truth*, New York: Semiotexte, pp. 41–82.

Fraser, N. (1989) *Unruly Practices: Power, Discourse, and Gender in Contemporary Social Theory*, Minneapolis, MN: University of Minnesota Press.

Habermas, J. (1990) *Moral Consciousness and Communication Interaction*, Cambridge: Polity Press.

Heidegger, M. (1962) *Being and Time*, Oxford: Wiley-Blackwell.

Kittay, Eva F. (1999) *Love's Labor: Essays on Women, Equality and Dependency*, New York: Routledge.

MacIntyre, A. (1985) *After Virtue: A Study in Moral Theory* (2nd edn), London: Duckworth.

Midgley, M. (2003) *Heart and Mind* (Revised edn), London: Routledge.

Murdoch, I. (1970) *The Sovereignty of Good*, London: Routledge.

Nichols, S. (2004) *Sentimental Rules: On the Natural Foundations of Moral Judgment*, Oxford: Oxford University Press.

Nussbaum, M. C. (2000) *Women and Human Development*, Cambridge: Cambridge University Press.

Nussbaum, M. C. (2001) *Upheavals of Thought: The Intelligence of Emotions*, Cambridge: Cambridge University Press.

O'Neill, J. (1994) Essentialism and markets, *The Philosophical Forum*, XXVI(2), 87–100.

Putnam, H. (2002) *The Collapse of the Fact-Value Dichotomy*, Cambridge, MA: Harvard University Press.

Rosaldo, R. (1989) *Culture and Truth*, London: Routledge.

Sayer, A. (2000a) *Realism and Social Science*, London: Sage.

Sayer, A. (2000b) For Postdisciplinary Studies: Sociology and the Curse of Disciplinary Parochialism/Imperialism. In Eldridge, J., MacInnes, J., Scott, S., Warhurst, C., & Witz, A. (eds.), *Sociology: Legacies and Prospects*, Durham: Sociology Press, pp. 85–97.

Sayer, A. (2006) Language and significance – Or the importance of import: Implications for critical discourse analysis, *Journal of Language and Politics*, 5(3), 449–471.

Sayer, A. (2011) *Why Things Matter to People: Social Science, Values and Ethical Life*, Cambridge: Cambridge University Press.

Sen, A. (1999) *Development as Freedom*, Oxford: Oxford University Press.

Shotton, L., & Seedhouse, D. (1998) Practical dignity in caring, *Nursing Ethics*, 5(3), 246–255.

Social Care Institute for Excellence (2013) www.scie.org.uk/publications/guides/guide15/

Soper, K. (1990) *Troubled Pleasures*, London: Verso.

Taylor, C. (1973) Neutrality and Political Science. In Ryan, A. (ed.), *The Philosophy of Social Explanation*, Oxford: Oxford University Press, pp. 139–170.

Taylor, C. (1985) *Philosophical Papers 1: Human Agency and Language*, Cambridge: Cambridge University Press.

Tronto, J. C. (1994) *Moral Boundaries*, London: Routledge.

Walzer, M. (1989) *Interpretation and Social Criticism*, Cambridge, MA: Harvard University Press.

Wilkinson, R., & Pickett, K (2011) *The Spirit Level: Why More Equal Societies Almost Always Do Better*, London: Allen Lane.

Williams, B. (1985) *Ethics and the Limits of Philosophy*, Oxford: Oxford University Press.

Workplace Dignity Institute, South Africa, www.tutsea.co.za/organisations/8670/workplace-dignity-institute

4 Interdisciplinary work in a critical realist perspective

Berth Danermark

Introduction

The introductory chapter emphasized that professionals and researchers both constantly encounter complex problems, which can be addressed in an interdisciplinary manner. Of course, this is a well-established insight; for instance, the US National Academy of Sciences Report (National Academy of Sciences, 2005) had an elegiac call for interdisciplinarity that described it as "one of the most productive and inspiring of human pursuits – one that provides a format for conversations and connections that lead to new knowledge . . . [and has] delivered much already and promises more – a sustainable environment, healthier and more prosperous lives, new discoveries and technologies to inspire young minds, and a deeper understanding of our place in space and time" (Ibid., 16). However, it has been shown that putting interdisciplinarity into practice is a demanding task. The aim of this chapter is to elaborate the challenging process of interdisciplinary work. Such a process goes through many phases. From being an expert in a certain field, such as social work, one collaborates with professionals from other fields; for instance, trained child psychiatrists and teachers. This multidisciplinary phase is characterized by cross-disciplinary understanding – for example, learning from each other. Cross-disciplinary learning is a precondition for the next phase of a successful interdisciplinarity work, which includes integrating the knowledge that all the members of the team have brought to the fore. This is the most crucial and challenging phase of interdisciplinary work. If it fails, the team will remain at a multidisciplinary level. If one reaches the point where the team has a broad understanding of the object, the last phase is to utilize the enlarged picture in a program for intervention.

This chapter addresses these different phases of interdisciplinary work; before proceeding, however, some clarifications need to be made. The first is what is meant in this chapter by "interdisciplinary work". This term refers to two types of activities: research and professional work. The former has a *scientific function* in which a deep understanding of a phenomenon that can answer questions about causality and making predictions are the core of the activities; for example, what are the causes of climate change and what will the future be like. The latter activity has a *transformative function*. One wishes to alter a non-desired state of affairs to a desired one – for example, reduce carbon dioxide emissions. There are many commonalities between interdisciplinary research and interdisciplinary teamwork among practitioners. The core and essence of the process is the same, but there are some differences that will be highlighted in the chapter.

The second clarification is related to what is meant by "interdisciplinary". In a review of the literature, Aboelela et al. (2007) identified some important aspects of interdisciplinary research: qualitatively different modes of research; a continuum of collaboration; fidelity to disciplinarity; increasing cooperation, communication and information sharing; and the epistemic status of the research outcome. The definition they proposed is as follows:

> Interdisciplinary research is any study or group of studies undertaken by scholars from two or more distinct scientific disciplines. The research is based upon a conceptual model that links or integrates theoretical frameworks from those disciplines, uses study design and methodology that is not limited to any one field, and requires the use of perspectives and skills of the involved disciplines throughout multiple phases of the research process.
>
> (Aboelela et al., 2007, p. 341)

There are at least two important distinctive features in this definition. It is a broad definition since only two disciplines need to be included to be considered inter-disciplinary work. In this chapter, I will treat interdisciplinary mainly in terms of a biopsychosocial approach that includes many disciplines or professions. The second feature of the definition is the emphasis on integration and that this should characterize the entire process. The definition emphasizes the integration of theo-retical frameworks. However, an important aspect that is not explicitly mentioned is the integration of the knowledge outcome of what each distinct discipline pro-duces; that is, integration of knowledge, not only theoretical frameworks. At the end of the chapter, I will come back to the question of definition and propose a modified version based on ontological insights from critical realism, which are missing in Aboelela et al.'s definition.

Why is interdisciplinarity necessary?

Although there is a growing awareness that interdisciplinarity has been shown to be the backbone of more or less all scientific breakthrough over the last 100 years, there is no consensus about how to philosophically approach interdisciplinary research and interdisciplinary professional practice. One line of argument is that it has been shown to produce fruitful knowledge that can lay the groundwork for successful interventions. This important epistemological argument is often seen in the literature (e.g. Frodeman, 2014; Newell, 2001; Kessel et al., 2008). From a critical realist perspective, however, there is a more fundamental argument for interdisciplinarity: it is a consequence of the *nature of the world*. Practically all events in real life occur in what are called open systems. In well-designed experi-ments, there is the possibility to more or less close the system, which means that one isolates the phenomenon one wishes to investigate so it cannot be affected by any factors other than those you are interested in. Then you manipulate it and register the outcome. This is seldom possible regarding human-related phenomenon. In real social life, there are mechanisms at different levels that influence the outcome, such as emergence, contradictions, and absence. This means that the core argument for interdisciplinary is ontological. This approach has been given many names, including holism, ecology, complex theory, and holistic causality (e.g. Bhaskar & Danermark, 2006; Høyer & Næss, 2008; Bhaskar et al., 2010; Holland, 2014; Price, 2014).

The introductory chapters of this book presented and discussed some basic ontological and epistemological concepts in critical realism, which will not be repeated here. It is necessary to have an understanding of these concepts when reading this chapter, although at some points it is necessary to further develop some of these concepts in the context of interdisciplinarity.

Why bother about ontology?

Interdisciplinary research involves many challenges – theoretical, methodological, individual, administrative, and financial (I will consider some of these below) – so why add another; namely, metatheoretical? The history of interdisciplinary research clearly illustrates that without a common understanding of the reality under investigation and a common agreement of epistemology, such as what is a legitimate scientific argument and what is not, there is a great risk that the process will end up failing to reach the goal of a bigger picture. For instance, if the research team includes persons with a strong affiliation to positivism and social constructivism, it is more likely that the integrative phase will not be reached due to basic divergent opinion on both ontology and epistemology. The process will at best end up at a multidisciplinary level. However, the most important reason for introducing a critical realist ontology is that it will guide the process toward an in-depth understanding of a complex phenomenon, avoiding eclecticism and reductionism.

In professional interdisciplinary work, such as multi-team work, there is also a need for a common metatheory ground, although it is seldom discussed explicitly in these terms. The American psychiatrist George Engel (1977; 1981) coined the concept biopsychosocial approach in health care. The background was his experiences of how professionals dealing with children and adolescents with psychiatric problems were not collaborating and that their ideas regarding how to cope with a psychiatric problem were sometimes contradictory and that their input caused more harm than help. We often see this kind of tension in social work and health care today. An example is the discussion about the extent to which a child's misbehavior is related to social conditions or to malfunctioning in the brain. Furthermore, there is a need in professional work to reach decisions regarding what kind of interventions should be made. This is based on factors such as resources in terms of money for and knowledge of different types of therapies, analysis of the causes of the actual condition, and experiences of outcomes of such intervention.

The discussion of evidence – based on practice, sometimes labeled knowledge-based practice – is an illustrative example of the importance of explicit metatheoretical discussions. The answer to the basic question of "what is evidence?" is always rooted in ontology, although the practitioner is sometimes not aware of his or her metatheoretical position.

The interdisciplinary process

In the first paragraph of this chapter, I indicated that the process of interdisciplinary work can be divided into different phases, as illustrated in Figure 4.1.

Before discussing each phase, some comments are necessary. First, the figure highlights what is an important and distinctive aspect of critical realism: namely, the disambiguation between ontology and epistemology. This has been dealt with in the previous chapters, but requires further explanation in the context of interdisciplinary work. In this context, disambiguation refers to the idea that there exists a reality "out there" that cannot be reduced to our understanding of it. In critical realist terms, there exists an intransitive dimension that is the object for the

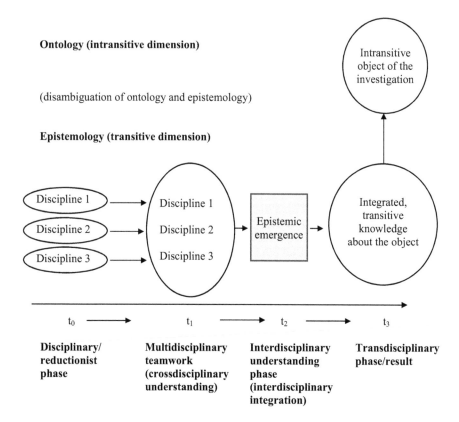

Figure 4.1 Four phases of interdisciplinary work

investigation or intervention, and a transitive dimension, which is our understanding of it. For instance, if a researcher or practitioner claims that his or her understanding of a phenomenon (the transitive dimension) is as true as another person's understanding, in short relativism, and if these understandings are contradictory, one ends up with real problems when doing interdisciplinary work.

The second point is that the four phases are in real life not as distinct as Figure 4.1 indicates. There is usually considerable overlap between the first three phases. However, it is worth making an analytical distinction between the phases.

Another important aspect, the third comment, is that there is always feedback. The outcome in one phase will impact the previous phase. For instance, it could be the case that new insights are gleaned during the cross-disciplinary learning, which leads to the discovery of structures and mechanisms that were not known in the first phase.

Structures, mechanisms, and emergence

Before discussing the different phases in detail, we must go back to what was said about mechanisms in Chapter 2. Mechanisms are things that can generate a change. It is a metaphorical term for a power by virtue of the structure of a phenomenon. Under certain conditions, this quality of being is triggered by something in the context and generates a change. An outcome is usually the result of a number of concurrent structures. For instance, if you perform an inappropriate action and become aware of it, you might blush at your mistake. The event of blushing can be understood as an interplay between biological structures (the superficial vessels widen), structures in the brain (autonomic nervous system), and norm structures (violating existing norms); in short, a biopsychosocial understanding. However, the potentiality to blush is always present, as a potentiality; sometimes it is triggered, sometimes it is not. Knowing that you will blush often makes it you blush more. This is an example of a reinforcing mechanism (knowledge). However, one can also create counteracting mechanisms, such as psychological mechanisms by cognitive therapy, or biological mechanisms such as beta-blockers or antidepressants.

The example illustrates that mechanisms are potentialities that can be manifested and even reinforced by other mechanisms, but they can also be counteracted so that there is no empirical manifestation.

We could say that we start with causes and move to structures and mechanisms, then to theories and end up with disciplines. The next step is to move to multidisciplinarity. The reason why we must deal with a multiplicity of disciplines is emergence. When one level of reality is emergent from another, it cannot be reduced to the lower level. An example of this is that an emotion cannot be reduced to chemical processes in the brain. It is emergent on the level of psychology. Therefore, we have to include different disciplines in the analysis.

By having the structure-mechanisms-event in unreducible levels (that is, emergence) in mind, it becomes clear that, in interdisciplinary work, in-depth knowledge of level-specific types of this triad is a precondition for an understanding of a complex phenomenon. In other words, one has to generate knowledge how different structures and mechanisms are operating at different strata. However, this is not sufficient. We also need to gain knowledge about how these different strata-specific mechanisms interact; this is the cross-disciplinary understanding. Being an expert on structure-mechanisms-event at certain strata and learning the interaction between different strata are the first two phases of the process of interdisciplinary, to which we now turn.

Phase 1: being an expert

Given that the world is constituted by open systems and that these systems – such as emotional, economic, and cultural – interact, experts are needed in each of these systems. Depending on which levels and which types of structures and mechanisms are involved, there is a need for people who know the state of the art in these levels. They have to be able to grasp the deep structure and find the mechanisms involved in producing the phenomenon, which is the object for the interdisciplinary work. These individuals must be trained in the discipline or the area of knowledge that is relevant and needed for a holistic understanding. For instance, if the object is the growing consumption of legally prescribed psychiatric drugs among children and adolescents, resulting in a substantial increase of deaths among that group, experts would be required in areas such as medicine, social work, political science, and jurisprudence. In this phase, each expert must move from the empirical manifested event to the structures and mechanisms that produce the event at the level he or she is an expert in. This requires in-depth knowledge of the possible explanatory mechanisms of the phenomenon. It also requires the skills to eliminate competing alternative explanations (given the actual context) and the outcome of this disciplinary phase is the most plausible explanation of which structures and mechanisms at a certain level are involved in the generating of the phenomenon. This is, in short, the disciplinary phase that all interdisciplinary processes must begin with.

This illustrates the point that the sometimes proposed contradiction between disciplinary work and interdisciplinary work is false. There have been claims that interdisciplinary research is not at the edge of science (see Rowe, 2008, p. 7), but, as described earlier, this is a misunderstanding based on the incorrect assumption that the interdisciplinary process does not incorporate the latest findings in an area of knowledge. On the contrary, it is truly at the edge since it will produce new knowledge about the interaction between mechanisms at different levels, information that a unidisciplinary approach will not be able to catch due to its reductionism.

A precondition for successful work is that the researchers and the practitioners involved are fully aware that their contributions at this stage of the process are only partial. Any claims *a priori* that this or that type of mechanisms are more important than mechanisms related to other levels of reality is a threat to the inter-disciplinary process. For instance, it is counterproductive to claim *a priori* that domestic violence is mainly caused by mental health problems, a lack of coping skills, substance abuse, gender relation, or religious mechanisms. At this phase of the process, the relative importance and role of different structures and mecha-nisms is still an open question.

In order to deepen the understanding of the interplay among all the iden-tified relevant mechanisms, one must move to the next phase, which is cross-disciplinary learning.

Phase 2: cross-disciplinary learning

Many of the obstacles for smooth interdisciplinary work at this phase can be sorted out by turning to the ontology of critical realism. Bhaskar has deepened the ontology of human beings as being reflexive and self-conscious, and in this context there are two aspects of his ontology that are more important than oth-ers. The first is the ability to understand that others have beliefs and perspectives that are different from one's own. The second aspect is that all human beings are learning beings.

In this phase, a number of different aspects of interdisciplinary work come to the fore. In a book on case studies of successful interdisciplinary research (Kessel et al., 2008), Rowe identified a number of determinants of success of interdisci-plinary research (see Rowe, 2008, pp. 5–8). Complementary skills is one of the investigator-specific factors, but this is related to the previous disciplinary phase. Another factor, which is an aspect of the cross-disciplinary phase, is the ability to develop a common language. This requires insight into other disciplines; that is, learning from each other. However, it is not just a question of understanding each other. In order to pave the way for creative interaction and problem solving among the researchers or practitioners, one researcher must learn from the other about which of the most important structures and mechanisms are related to other levels than the one that the first researcher is an expert in. Of course, it is not a question of being an expert in the other's field, but it is necessary to get a basic understanding of other disciplines.

This always triggers a number of aspects other than the cognitive in the pro-cess of interdisciplinary work. The most obvious may be the interactive aspects. Hence, Rowe (2008) mentioned the need for "true openness to the approaches, perspectives, and attitudes of scientists from other disciplines" (p. 6). A number of studies (e.g. Sawa, 2005; Pohl, 2005; Stokols et al., 2005) have shown, for instance, that the encounter of researchers or practitioners in an interdiscipli-nary team is characterized by what Jovchelovitch (2007) called the domination approach (the opposite of a dialogical approach). In this context, the domination approach means that one expert, researcher, or practitioner claims that his or her perspective and understanding of a phenomenon should be the one dominating the process and that others in the team should embrace that, while the dialogical approach means a true openness for other perspectives.

This situation can be dealt with by the *critical realist embrace*. This means that critical realism is the metatheory that can epistemologically include important insights from various other metatheories.

> It acknowledges the importance of a) the descriptive moment in the natural sciences, which is the moment associated with measuring things and carrying out experiments; b) the neo-Kantian moment which is the retroductive moment associated with the identification of a generative structure; c) the point at which we must eliminate alternative theories; and then d) the point at which we come back to an empirical moment.
>
> (Bhaskar et al., 2018, p. 82)

This paves the way for a dialogical approach.

Furthermore, a dialogical approach includes mutual respect for researchers and practitioners from fields other than one's own as an important aspect of interdisciplinary work. Respect is most often based on at least a basic understanding and knowledge of the mainstream theories and methodologies and other conditions that influence the approach by other members of the team. Hence, non-respect is the outcome of ignorance. An illustrative example is a study among Canadian biomedical scientists, which found a predominantly negative attitude toward the social sciences (Albert et al., 2008). The main reason for not viewing social science as scientific was that its methods did not conform to experimental designs. It is important to note that those respondents who were negative had no experiences of collaborations with social scientists. The study indicates that their negative attitude was based, among other things, on ignorance of social science methods. Those with experiences and insights into the methods used in the social sciences were more positive.

Beside this methodological hierarchy, another reason for disrespect is the hierarchy that exists among disciplines and professions (for a discussion on this topic, see Danermark & Germundsson, 2011).

Phase 3: integrating knowledge

After the first two phases, we should have from each discipline or area of knowledge in-depth knowledge about the structures and mechanisms that are relevant in relation to the complex phenomenon under study. We should also have participants in the research team or professional team who have good insights into the other areas of knowledge that are involved. In this third phase, the challenges of knowledge integration will come to the fore. There are no strict procedures to follow in this phase. It is a stage where flourishing creativity is the driving force; a creativity fertilized by the true interaction among the members of the team. This process, as Bhaskar (2010) emphasized, "proceeds by a basic procedure involving the identification and correction of mistakes" (p. 19). Critique and reflexive self-critique is a salient feature of this activity. Therefore, it is extremely important that the cross-disciplinary learning phase is characterized by mutual respect and openness for influences from other disciplines. This transformation of thinking can, at one extreme, take the form of transformative learning, which Elias (1997) defined as "the expansion of consciousness through the transformation of basic worldview and specific capacities of the self; transformative learning is facilitated through consciously directed processes such as appreciatively accessing and receiving the symbolic contents of the unconscious and critically analyzing underlying premises" (p. 3). However, not all learning is transformative. Mezirow & Associates (2000) posited that there is a difference between transmissional, transactional, and transformational forms of learning. Transmissional learning is characterized by the fact that it is "transmitted" from one person in the team to another. It is incorporated in the knowledge of the receiving person, but it does not alter any views of the subject for research or professional collaboration in any significant way. It might only give further support for a certain view. The second type of learning, transactional, occurs through experience, inquiry, critical thinking, and interaction with other members of the team, and it might have some impact on the person's understanding. Brookfield (2000) argued that learning could only be transformative if it involves an in-depth critical reflection of taken-for-granted assumptions. For many "hard core" discipline-oriented researchers or professionals, the experiences of being involved in truly interdisciplinary work could sometimes result in transformative learning. This transformative praxis is further developed in Bhaskar's dialectical critical realism (e.g. Bhaskar, 2008).

As mentioned previously, there are no strict guidelines for knowledge integration. Danermark et al. (2002) and Bhaskar et al., 2018) provide some general guidelines based on what Bhaskar (2008) calls the RRREI(C) schema. This schema is applied in the context when scientists are concerned with *explaining events that happen in the open systemic world.*

R_1 stands for the *resolution* of the complex phenomenon into its components, involving a conjunctive multiplicity of causes (that is, a *and* b *and* c, etc.); R_2 for the abductive *redescription* or recontextualisation of these components in an explanatorily significant way; R_3 for the *retrodiction* of these component causes to antecedently existing events or states of affairs; E for the *elimination* of alternative competing explanatory antecedents; I for the *identification* of the causally efficacious antecedent (or antecedent complex); and C for the iterative *correction* of earlier findings in the light of this (albeit provisionally) completed explanation or analysis.

However, if the outcome of this process leads us to conclude that we have *not* been able to identify the underlying structure and mechanisms that cause the observed phenomenon and we are facing anomalies, we must turn to Bhaskar's DREI(C)[1] model of pure science, which contains the logic of *theory building*. It is a "creative process in which the researcher arrives at something new, perhaps even surprising, to better account for the empirical evidence" (Bhaskar et al., 2018). That means we are looking for a key creative moment that leads to the new theory. This phase of developing a new theory outlines the basic structures and mechanisms (for a concrete illustration, see an example of research on the epidemiology of HIV in Africa by Price, 2010).

However, this suggestion for guidelines should not be confused with what Frodeman (2014) called "Methodism," which means applying methodological prescriptions that act as straitjackets. Critical realists embrace the idea of methodological pluralism and specificity. It is important that the interdisciplinary research is theory-driven, not method-driven (Danermark, 2002b).

These general guidelines can also be applied in professional work. For instance, if one encounters a problem such as school bullying, the overall process could be the same: describe bullying in all its components in a certain context, identify programs for dealing with school bullying, eliminate those programs that are not knowledge-based and choose the one that seems most likely to fit into the actual context, investigate the circumstances that seem to have triggered the bullying at the school and, based on that, implement a tailored program and evaluate and make corrections if necessary.

However, there is one crucial element in this phase that needs to be further developed. This is the application of a laminated system – that is, including all the relevant levels of reality in the investigation or the implementation of a social program.

Necessary laminated systems

In order to avoid fragmentation, reductionism, and oversimplification, the interdisciplinary research team or the multi-professional team must include all the relevant levels of reality in their understanding of a phenomenon – that is, construct a laminated system consisting of a conjunctive multiplicity of levels of reality. Bhaskar and Danermark (2006) argued that this should even be called "a *necessarily* laminated system" since there are levels that cannot be excluded in the analysis or the intervention unless the understanding of the phenomenon or the alteration of it will be severely hampered. For instance, if a social program that aims to reduce drug abuse focuses solely on the supply side, neglecting the demand side, it is doomed to fail. In research, one cannot successfully investigate an issue such as anorexia nervosa without taking the social level into account, such as the thinness culture in media.

An important question for a team to answer is: What levels need to be included in the analysis? The answer must be guided by a pragmatic view related to the aim of the study and the endeavor of the multidisciplinary professional teamwork. There are a number of examples of constructing a necessarily laminated system that can serve as illustrations (see Bhaskar et al., 2018). One of the first examples, based on a critical realist ontology and epistemology, was presented by Bhaskar and Danermark (2006). The example was related to disability and the underlying question was, "How can we understand a phenomenon such as disability without committing the fallacy of reductionism?" Their answer was that an analysis of disability should consist of seven levels including mechanisms, types of context, and characteristic effects. These levels are: (1) physical, (2) biological (more specifically, physiological, medical, or clinical), (3) psychological, (4) psychosocial, (5) socio-economic, (6) cultural, and (7) normative (ibid., pp. 288–289). Another example of construction of a laminated system is related to education and learning (Brown, 2009), whose five levels were: (1) biological mechanisms, such as adequate nutrition; (2) physical mechanisms, such as classroom lighting; (3) psychological mechanisms, such as student motivation; (4) sociocultural (including moral and political) mechanisms, such as parental beliefs about education; and (5) normative mechanisms, as determined by curricula. The two previous examples are rooted in critical realism, but there are a number of examples in science that are based on an idea of levels of reality, although these are not explicitly anchored in critical realism. A well-known example is George Engels' aforementioned biopsychosocial model for analyzing psychiatric disorders using General System Theory (GST) (Engels, 1977). Another similar theoretical approach is Urie Bronfenbrenner's Ecological System Theory (EST) (Bronfenbrenner, 1979). In short, the outcome of the work with creating a laminated system is an *integrative analytic tool*.

Four-planar system

The next step in interdisciplinary studies is to include what Bhaskar called the four-planar system (Bhaskar, 2008, Chapter 2.9). In this system, every social event "can be understood in terms of four dimensions, namely: (1) material transactions with nature, (2) social interactions between agents, (3) social structure proper, and (4) the stratification of embodied personalities of agents" (Bhaskar & Danermark, 2006). This means that more or less all activities have a relation to nature (for example, when driving a car there is an impact on the environment); that social activities are performed in relation to other people and are taking place in a social context with a certain social structure; and that the biopsychosocial history of a person is important. This concept was developed into a "Research map" by Layder (1993, p. 72), who suggested that the research map should include four basic research elements. The first is self, which includes self-identity and the individual's social experience. The second is situated activity; that is, social activity such as face-to-face activity involving symbolic communication by skilled, intentional participants implicated in the above contexts and settings. This element involves a focus on emergent meanings, understandings, and definitions of the situation as these affect and are affected by contexts and settings and subjective dispositions of individuals. The third element is setting; for example, intermediate social organizations such as labor markets, hospitals, social work agencies, domestic labor, and organization of leisure activities and religious organizations. The fourth and final element is the context of a macro social organization, which includes phenomena such as values, traditions, and forms of social and economic organization and power relations.

How to practice interdisciplinarity?

A common and pertinent question is how to *practice* interdisciplinary research. As indicated in the previous paragraphs, the rule of thumb is to use methods that are developed for the respective level – that is, methodological specificity. It is important to consider how different methodologies can lead to knowledge about generative mechanisms. The way in which different levels of reality are methodologically approached is determined by the scope of openness. For instance, experiment can be applied if there is a possibility to close the system; in other cases, quasi experiments can be relevant, but when it comes to the social level, other methods must be applied, such as in-depth interviews and observations. However, such methodological plurality must be guided by ontology; if not, there is a risk of unprincipled eclecticism, which we sometimes see under the name of mixed methodologies. Different methodological approaches are usually described in terms of quantitative and qualitative methods, respectively. Another dichotomy – intensive and extensive – is described in Danermark et al. (2002, chapter 7). In the search for generative mechanisms and how they can explain events in various contexts, one can distinguish between these two empirical procedures, whereas "the intensive empirical procedure contains substantial parts of data collecting and analyses of a qualitative kind. The extensive procedure has to do with quantitative data-collecting and statistical analysis" (p. 163). It is important to emphasize that the first mentioned procedure focuses on generative mechanisms by tracing the causal power and the interaction between powers that produce a social phenomenon. However, in order to find out the frequencies of a certain phenomenon, what characteristics it has, and other empirical manifestations, one must turn to extensive designs. Moreover, a certain mechanism does not manifest itself randomly in real life. As Lawson (1997) wrote, "Over restricted regions of time-space certain mechanisms may come to dominate others and/or shine through", and these mechanisms are "giving rise to rough and ready generalities or partial generalities, holding to such a degree that *prima facie* an explanation is called for" (p. 204). The history of social science clearly shows how some of these mechanisms that Lawson called demi-regularities are very stable, such as gender, class, and ethnicity patterns.

This interdisciplinary teamwork phase can be summarized by stating that an analysis of a complex phenomenon includes the relevant levels. Which levels to include must be decided in relation to the objective of the research. At each relevant level, one should identify the most important structures, the mechanisms they generate, and the events produced by these mechanisms using the theories, research designs (both intensive and extensive designs), and methods that are developed for the respective level.

Phase 4: interventions – the acid test

We have now reached a point where we have a broader picture that it is hoped covers all relevant levels with their structures and mechanisms. We also have knowledge about the interactions between these mechanisms, which enables us to understand and explain the phenomenon. This integrated understanding is the point of departure in this phase.

As mentioned at the beginning of this chapter, most research and professional work is directed toward a problem that one wishes to transform to a less problematic condition, or even better, totally eliminate the problem. This is done by different forms of intervention that intend to make things better. Not all interdisciplinary research processes take this final step; in most cases, however, the knowledge produced by an interdisciplinary research team is used in different forms of interventions, if not by the research team itself, by other actors. In professional work the *raison d'être* is often intervention. These interventions are sometimes labeled "social programs". From a critical realist point of view, these interventions can take different forms. They can focus on *changing the structure* that gives rise to mechanisms and hence the outcomes, or they can *create counteracting mechanisms* to reduce the negative outcome. They can also *support mechanisms* that result in positive outcome. All three types of activities presuppose knowledge that is based on interdisciplinary work; that is, a necessarily laminated system. In real life, these different forms of interventions interact and can be implemented simultaneously. For instance, creating counteracting mechanisms can change the structure in the long run.

Changing the structure

Changing the underlying structure is the most radical way of intervention, although it is often difficult to achieve in a short-term perspective. The potential for an intervention to change underlying structures is illustrated by the example of child abuse (beating). In Sweden, child abuse was considered a social problem, rather than an individual problem, in the 1960s and 1970s. Research clearly demonstrated the negative aspects of child abuse. Sixty years of research has not been able to demonstrate a positive outcome of child abuse, but it has shown a number of negative outcomes (Gershoff, 2002). One of the most important underlying structures was the norm structure, which included the norm of punishment related to all forms of misbehavior of the child. This norm was very established (and still is in many countries). In 1979, in an attempt to change this norm structure, the Swedish government was the first in the world to pass a law prohibiting child abuse. In critical realist terms, the government created a counteracting mechanism. This did not alter the norm structure in the short term but, after some decades, it has changed and the prevailing norm in Sweden is currently extremely negative regarding child abuse. This is also a global trend. As of 2016, approximately fifty countries have now prohibited all types of child abuse, both domestic and outside the family.

Making predictions

In this section, I will argue for the theory/practice ensemble by emphasizing a close connection among explanations, intervention, and predictions anchored in the ontology and epistemology of critical realism.

In the social world, intervention is closely related to the possibility to make predictions. One must legitimize an intervention in terms of its predicted outcome – that is, predict the result of the intervention. Making predictions is often seen as a criterion of a good and mature science, but making predictions is an extremely challenging task. In the open social world, such as macroeconomics, it is notorious how often predictions fail. Based on a critical realist ontology, the question is whether it is possible to make trustworthiness predictions in open systems (Sayer, 1992; Lawson, 1997).

In closed systems, the acting mechanisms always produce the same result, but the outcomes in open systems vary. In critical realism, this can lead to a position that we can call explanatory non-predictive (Danermark et al., 2002, p. 183). However, despite the open character of the social world, it is possible to make reliable predictions. Bhaskar (1978, p. 68) stated that many things are de facto predictable. In this vein, a number of critical realists over the last decade have presented a more positive view on predictions (Næss, 2004; Karlsson, 2009; Næss & Strand, 2012). Næss (2004) argued that it is possible, to some extent, to make predictions, but one cannot make accurate predictions of future *events* or *situations*. He concluded that predictions from a critical realist perspective can be made regarding aggregate-scale main tendencies, but not the actions of individuals.

He argued that the possibility to make predictions should not be confused with positivist, actualist, and reductionist standardized methods based on, for example, randomized controlled trials (RCT), which some believe are the gold standard practice for claiming evidence-based practice and hence predictions. At best, a method such as RCT is just one piece in the puzzle. By itself, it cannot answer why a certain intervention produced a certain outcome and hence be the foundation for accurate predictions in different social contexts.

Important in the discussion about prediction is the question of whether open and closed systems are a dichotomy – that is, a system is either closed or opened. Alternatively, it can be understood as a scale with total closeness and total openness at the two ends of the scale. There is no consensus among critical realists on this issue. On the one hand, because social systems are inhabited by human beings who are reflexive and creative, all such systems are open. On the other hand, due to the same human virtue, people can act in a way that counteracts mechanisms that are "opening the system" (Karlsson, 2009) – that is, creating a more or less open system. Those who argue that there is a qualitative difference between open and closed systems tend to be reluctant to affirm the possibility of making predictions in the social world, while those who see it as "more or less" seem to be more positive about the possibility of making predictions. I would argue that critical realism provides us with knowledge that makes it possible to make reliable predictions, but this requires an interdisciplinary approach. It is an empirical observation that demi-regularities exist, although these regularities are quasi-stable and only partly predictable. The explanation of the existence of demi-regularities are long-term, enduring social structures. People are reflexive and creative, but they often act in such a way that these structures are reproduced by acting habitual behavior (habitus to speak with Bourdieu, 1984) and intentionally or unconsciously upholding a social or cultural structure. These structures can also be stable due to power relations; for example, the economic global interest in the oil industry, which prevents nations from acting according to climate agreements despite having signed and ratified the agreements.

In short, a precondition for making predictions in the social world is that the structures that have been identified in the interdisciplinary work are rather stable. Economic, gender, class, and ethnic structures are examples of such long-term and rather stable structures.

Some degree of "event regularity" (such as in the occurrence and strength of mechanisms pulling in a certain direction compared to the occurrence and strength of counteracting mechanisms) at a lower stratum is a precondition for the emergence of a structure at a higher stratum. For example, a more frequent occurrence of neoliberal political beliefs than opposing beliefs in the population may lead to a parliamentary election resulting in a more neoliberal political structure on a national scale. In some cases, the emergence of causal relationships at a higher ontological stratum presupposes the existence of some "event regularity" at a lower stratum (Næss, 2016).

The point is to emphasize that any intervention in social life is better off being based on an in-depth critical realist guided interdisciplinary analysis. This has been illustrated by, for instance, Pawson and Tilly (1997) in their work on critical realist evaluation. Blom and Morén (2010) developed and applied a conceptual framework and a theoretical model for explaining the outcome of interventions in social work; that is, the results can be reconstructed *ex post* as conforming to critical realist schema. Although they do not explicitly discuss predictions, their approach and outcome of studies based on their model can be used for predictions.

Næss's claims about prediction are very modest. Elsewhere (Danermark, 2002b), it is argued that it is sometimes possible to give a reliable answer the question of what works for whom in what circumstances? This involves going a step further than Næss, who limited the possibility to predict aggregate-scale main tendencies, not the actions of individuals. I would argue that it is possible to make at least approximate predictions on the individual level regarding actions and other forms of outcomes of interventions. Predicting the outcome at the individual level is often the case in medicine and many other fields, such as social work and pedagogy; given that such predictions are based on a *correct explicit ex ante metatheory* and intensive interdisciplinary research strategy (Bhaskar & Danermark, 2006), they can be very accurate.

Summary

Danermark (2002a) provided a short and simplified definition: "interdisciplinary research is to study how a complex phenomenon is manifested at different levels" (p. 4). This definition refers to ontology, but it needs to be further developed.

A tentative critical realist informed definition is as follows: Interdisciplinary research is any study or group of studies undertaken by scholars from *all relevant levels* that are needed to answer the research question. The research is *integrating analysis of structures, mechanisms, and outcomes* at these levels by using *study design and methodology that are most appropriate for respective levels.* The output is *knowledge emergence*, which requires the use of skills of the involved researchers throughout multiple phases of the research process.

The highlights in this definition are levels, structures, mechanisms, outcome, methodological specificity, and knowledge emergence.

The definition can be unpacked by presenting seven aspects of interdisciplinary work discussed in this chapter (these aspects are discussed at length in Bhaskar et al., 2018), as follows:

i   The need for disambiguation, and in particular, to distinguish between ontology (intransitive dimension of science) and epistemology (transitive dimension of science);

ii   The idea of "levels of reality" implying a firm anchorage in certain fields of knowledge which are sometimes equal to disciplines, and sometimes not;

iii   The idea that the most appropriate methodological design differs between levels of reality;

iv   The conviction that a reductionist perspective is ontologically wrong and scientifically and practically unacceptable;

v   The idea of a laminated system with the corresponding insistence on the importance of knowledge in other areas besides one's own, as a condition for creativity in interdisciplinary research;

vi   Respect for the necessity and autonomy of metatheory and metatheoretical issues. Such issues are abstract and cannot be immediately and unequivocally coupled with empirical statements, without committing the fallacy of misplaced concreteness; and

vii   The idea of cross-disciplinary understanding and interdisciplinary and interprofessional integration as prerequisites for interdisciplinary research and interprofessional cooperation alike.

To conclude, interdisciplinary work based on a strategy of focusing on theories of structures and generative mechanisms will enable us to do three things. *First*, we will be able to better understand which mechanisms produce the changes a program has accomplished. *Second*, we will be able to increase our understanding of the contextual conditions that have to be at hand to let the mechanisms produce the wanted effects. *Third*, we will have an idea about the mechanisms and the context that enables us to make predictions of the outcome pattern and/or to better understand and interpret the outcome.

Note

1 DREI(C) is a model of pure scientific explanation. When we identify a problem, we resolve it into its components (description, D) and then we re-describe (R) it using the appropriate language. We then explain (E) it, by retrodiction, and thus gain an understanding of its antecedent causes (identifying, I) and, if necessary, make corrections (C).

References

Aboelela, S. W., Larson, E., Bakken, S., Olveen, C., Formicola, A., Glied, S. A., Haas, J., & Gebbie, K. M. (2007) Defining interdisciplinary research: Conclusions from a critical review of the literature, *Health Research and Educational Trust*, 42(1), Part I, 329–346.

Albert, M., Laberge, S., Hodges, B. D., Regehr, G., & Lingard, L. (2008) Biomedical scientists' perception of the social sciences in health research, *Social Science & Medicine*, 66, 2520–2531.

Bhaskar, R. (1978) *A Realist Theory of Science*, Hassocks: Harvester Press.

Bhaskar, R. (2008) *Dialectic: The Pulse of Freedom*, London: Routledge, Taylor & Francis.

Bhaskar, R. (2010) Contexts of Interdisciplinarity. In Bhaskar, R., Frank, C., Høyer, K. G., Naess, P., & Parker, J. (eds.), *Interdisciplinarity and Climate Change: Transforming Knowledge and Practice for Our Global Future*, New York: Routledge, pp. 2–24.

Bhaskar, R., & Danermark, B. (2006) Metatheory, interdisciplinarity and disability research: A critical realist perspective, *Scandinavian Journal of Disability Research*, 8(4), 278–297.

Bhaskar, R., Danermark, B., & Price, L. (2018) *Interdisciplinary and Wellbeing: A Critical Realist General Theory of Interdisciplinarity,* London: Routedge.

Bhaskar, R., Frank, C., Høyer, K. G., Naess, P., & Parker, J. (eds.) (2010) *Interdisciplinarity and Climate Change: Transforming Knowledge and Practice for Our Global Future*, New York: Routledge.

Blom, B., & Morén, S. (2010) Explaining social work practice – The CAIMeR theory, *Journal of Social Work*, 10(1), 98–119.

Bourdieu, P. (1984) *Distinction: A Social Critique of the Judgement of Taste*, Cambridge, MA: Harvard University Press.

Bronfenbrenner, U. (1979) *The Ecology of Human Development*, Cambridge, MA: Harvard University Press.

Brookfield, S. D. (2000) Transformative Learning as Ideology Critique. In Mezirow, J. & Associates (eds.), *Learning as Transformation: Critical Perspectives on a Theory in Progress*, San Francisco, CA: Jossey-Bass, pp. 125–150.

Brown, G. (2009) The Ontological Turn in Education: the Place of the Learning Environment, *Journal of Critical Realism*, 8(1), 5–34.

Danermark, B. (2002a) Interdisciplinary research and critical realism: The example of disability research, *International Journal of Critical Realism*, 5(1), 56–64.

Danermark, B. (2002b) Different approaches in assessment: A meta theoretical perspective, *International Journal of Audiology*, 42(Suppl 1), 112–117.

Danermark, B., Ekström, M., Jakobson, L., & Karlsson, J. (2002) *Explaining Society: Critical Realism in the Social Sciences,* London: Routledge.

Danermark, B., & Germundsson, P. (2011) Social Representation and Power. Chapter 2. In Chaib, M., Danermark, B., & Selander, S. (eds.), *Education, Professionalization and Social Representations: On the Transformation of Social Knowledge*, London: Routledge, 33–43.

Elias, D. (1997) It's time to change our minds: An introduction to transformative learning, *ReVision*, 20(1), 2–6.

Engel, G. (1977) The need for a new medical model: A challenge for biomedicine, *Science*, 196, 129–136.

Engel, G. (1981) The clinical application of the biopsychosocial model, *Journal of Medicine and Philosophy*, 6, 101–123.

Frodeman, R. (2014) *Sustainable Knowledge: A Theory of Interdisciplinarity*, New York: Palgrave Macmillan.

Gershoff, E. T. (2002) Corporal punishment by parents and associated child behaviors and experiences: A meta-analytic and theoretical review, *Psychol Bull*, 128(4), 539–579, doi:10.1037/0033–2909.128.4.539.

Holland, G. (2014) *Integrating Knowledge Through Interdisciplinary Research: Problems of Theory and Practice*, London: Routledge.

Høyer, K. G., & Naess, P. (2008) Interdisciplinary, ecology and scientific theory: the case of sustainable urban development, *Journal of Critical Realism*, 7(2), 179–207.

Jovchelovitch, S. (2007) *Knowledge in Context: Representations, Community and Culture*, London: Routledge.

Karlsson, J. Ch. (2009) Delvis öppna och delvis slutna system [Partly Open and Partly Closed Systems]. In Bengtsson, M., Daoud, A., & Seldén, D. (eds.), *En realistisk sociologi i praktiken. Nio texter om samhället [A realist sociology in practice. Nine texts about society]*, *Research report no. 141*, Gothenburg: Department of Sociology, University of Gothenburg, pp. 33–50.

Kessel, F., Rosenfield, P. L., & Anderson, N. B. (eds.) (2008) *Interdisciplinary Research: Case Studies From Health and Social Science*, New York: Oxford University Press.

Lawson, T. (1997) *Economics and Reality*, London: Routledge.

Layder, D. (1993) *New Strategies in Social Research: An Introduction and Guide*, Cambridge: Polity Press.

Mezirow, J., & Associates (eds.) (2000) *Learning as Transformation; Critical Perspectives on a Theory in Progress*, San Francisco, CA: Jossey-Bass, 125–150.

Næss, P. (2004) Prediction regressions and critical realism, *Journal of Critical Realism*, 3, 133–164.

Næss, P. (2016) Built environment, causality and urban planning, *Planning Theory & Practice*, 52–71, http://dx.doi.org/10.1080/14649357.2015.11277994.

Næss, P., & Strand, A. (2012) What kinds of traffic forecasts are possible? *Journal of Critical Realism*, 11(3), 277–295.

National Academy of Sciences (2004) *Facilitating Interdisciplinary Research: Committee on Science, Engineering, and Public Policy*, Washington, DC: National Academies Press.

Newell, W. (2001) A theory of interdisciplinary studies, *Issues in Integrative Studies*, 19, 1–25.

Pawson, R., & Tilly, N. (1997) *Realistic Evaluation*, London: Sage.

Pohl, C. (2005) Transdisciplinary collaboration in environmental research, *Futures*, 37, 1159–1178.

Price, L. (2010) The carnivalesque factor in southern African HIV pandemic, *Exchange on HIV/AIDS, Sexuality and Gender*, 2, 3–7.

Price, L. (2014) Critical realist versus mainstream interdisciplinarity, *Journal of Critical Realism*, 13(1), 52–76.

Rowe, J. W. (2008) Introduction: Approaching Interdisciplinary Research. In Kessel, F., Rosenfield, P. L., & Anderson, N. B. (eds.), *Expanding the Boundaries of Health and Social Science: Case Studies in Interdisciplinary Innovation*, Oxford: Oxford University Press, pp. 3–9.

Sawa, R. J. (2005) Foundations of interdisciplinarity, *Medicine, Health Care and Philosophy*, 8, 53–61.

Sayer, A. (1992) *Method in Social Science: A Realist Approach*, London: Routledge.

Stokols, D., Harvey, R., Gress, J., Fuqua, J., & Philips, K. (2005) In vivo studies of transdisciplinary scientific collaboration, *American Journal of Preventive Medicine*, 28, 202–213.

5 Learning to *absent* the absent

Critical realism and social work education

Stanley Houston and Lorna Montgomery

Introduction

There has been a growing interest in Roy Bhaskar's (1978; 1993; 1998) critical realism, and its contribution to social work, even though little has been written on the subject. The challenge of making the former more pertinent to the latter may lie in Bhaskar's use of technical terms, neologisms and acronyms when presenting his ideas. Another barrier is that philosophy can be viewed as an arcane subject for social work: one that is difficult to apply in practical, real-life circumstances. Yet, social workers practice in a world of ever-increasing complexity and oppression. Critical realism has so much to offer in this context, because it can act as an *under labourer* (Locke, 1700/1979) to the profession; that is, it winnows away the kernels of misapprehension, bringing a clear-sighted awareness of the causes of human suffering.

If there is merit in this proposition, the quintessential question at this point can be articulated as follows: how can critical realism be introduced to social workers in a meaningful way that enables them to apply its philosophical tenets with confidence? Relatedly, how can social work educators, at undergraduate and postgraduate levels, realise the potential of this body of thought and convey it adroitly to students in the classroom? Last, how can social workers extrapolate their (critical realist) learning to the social world to tackle oppression and promote transformative practice aimed at enhancing the well-being of service users?

In this chapter, I will tackle these questions by arguing that the key tenets of critical realism can be adeptly conveyed in the classroom and skilfully applied through problem-based learning (Clouston et al., 2010). This enabling approach is student-centred and organised around andragogical principles (Knowles et al., 2005). Andragogy recognises the centrality of the adult learner, where percipience comes about through self-reflection and group-based inquiry. Here, education is seen as investigative and propelled by an ineluctable curiosity. Such learning principles are most compatible with critical realism which seeks to encourage critical questioning, insights into causality and, most important, transformative praxis aimed at either removing or alleviating social injustice.

To consider this area in a structured way, I will first consider a number of key sources applying critical realism to social work. Overall, not much has been written on the subject from an educational stance. Thus, my intention is to show that a critical gap exists in our understanding of how critical realism can be introduced to social work students, whether in higher education settings or in other learning sites. Having presented the rationale for this inquiry, I will then outline what I consider to be the essential tenets of critical realism that social work students need to know if they are to adopt its perspective of the social world and the oppression that lies therein. As part of this elucidation, I will consider Bhaskar's work (1993) on *dialectical change*, a treatise that has received very little attention by the social work academy but nonetheless has considerable ramifications for emancipatory practice. This will then lead to an introduction to problem-based learning and, finally, an attempt to utilize it as a crucial method for making critical realism accessible to social work students.

A review of key sources

The existing literature (written in the English language) on critical realism and social work can be divided into three broad areas, namely: (a) research applications, (b) practice considerations and (c) epistemological (or knowledge-based) reflections. Although the sources within these areas do not consider how to educate social workers on the theme of critical realism, they provide a necessary resource for social work students seeking to understand the philosophy and apply it within problem-based learning.

Regarding research applications, in a previous publication (Houston, 2010) I made the case for adopting critical realism in qualitative approaches to data acquisition and analysis. Specifically, the article suggested that there was a concordance between critical realist premises and action research with its cyclical inquiry and advancement of social change. I contended that the combination of critical realist principles and action-oriented method provided a framework for anti-oppressive social work research. On further reflection, action research can be viewed as a form of problem-based learning given that it encourages a group-based analysis of presenting challenges, how to respond to them, and finally evaluate the outcomes of such endeavours.

Oliver (2012) has also made a convincing case for applying critical realism within qualitative research. In her view, critical realism is harmonious with recent attempts to rework grounded theory in ways that enable the method to take stock of the socially constructed nature of the social world; move beyond induction as the primary research orientation; and inquire critically into the interplay between agency and structure. With these modifications in place, Oliver argues that grounded theory can assimilate the critical realist approach of *retroduction*: a way of reasoning systematically about why events happen in the way that they do. (Later on in this chapter, I will explain the notion of retroduction more fully and integrate it within the stages of problem-based learning). Overall, Oliver's contribution is useful in that it argues that middle-range theory should build from not only empirical observation and surface description but also the causal level of unseen mechanisms. As has been argued elsewhere (Houston, 2005; Craig & Bigby, 2015), realist-informed qualitative methods should be seen as part of an evidence-informed paradigm of social work inquiry.

One other research-related application needs to be considered in addition those presented above. It sets out Longhofer and Floersch's (2014) impassioned plea for a 'values-informed' social work research. Drawing on a critical realist approach to ethics, they reject the 'fact-value' distinction and argue that social work practice and research are inherently normative. Thus, ethics ought to be centre stage in all inquiry. The 'ought' is what matters most to people as do people themselves; and the social act, whatever its nature, is rarely value-free. The salience of ethics in social work research applies also to social work education where students must be afforded the space and time to cogitate on complex value-dilemmas, including how to juxtapose care and control responses in an increasingly regulated profession.

The second area, categorised earlier as 'practice considerations', has generated a few written outputs most notable of which is Blom and Moren's (2010) inventive CAIMeR Theory. This contribution to knowledge amounts to a conceptual framework examining how outcomes in social work arise from various contingent factors: situational contexts, actors, interventions and results. Moreover, the theory is animated by critical realist ideas that specifically address the role of generative mechanisms at different levels, and how they create an understanding of both the 'how' and the 'why' of change: prising open the 'black box', as it were. Unfortunately, the authors only make a brief reference to social work education. This is a lost opportunity as the theory is comprehensive and schematically sophisticated.

The third categorisation centres on epistemology in social work. Mäntysaari (2005) poses a rhetorical question under this rubric: 'can a philosophical position called realism act as a foundation for social work knowledge in the three applications of social work: research, education and practice'? In response to this question, he argues that the antimony between objectivism and subjectivism in social research can be resolved through adopting a realist stance on knowledge production. This is because it respects objective causation and subjective meaning. Mäntysaari's stance chimes with Longhofer and Floersch's (2012) concerns regarding a knowledge crisis in social work. For the latter, critical realism is the solution to this crisis because it transcends the limitations of positivism and conventionalism in social work: two methodological perspectives that, they argue, have truncated knowledge production in social work.

The afore-mentioned valorisation of critical realism in these sources, while not directly addressing the theme of social work education, is nonetheless important for students. Indubitably, they need to know about the structural constraints shaping social work interventions (Briar-Lawson, 2012) including those arising from neoliberal contradictions in society (Houston, 2012).

Key tenets of critical realism for social work students

Critical realism is a philosophical perspective which provides an explanation of how complex mechanisms co-mingle in the social world to produce often unpredictable events. Given this emphasis, it has great relevance for social workers who need to understand causation when assessing and intervening in multi-faceted situations involving child and adult trauma. In this section, I highlight the central tenets of Bhaskar's critical realism (1978; 1993; 1998), those which I consider most apt for a problem-based learning approach geared toward social workers' learning and development. This summary is broken down into various parts, namely: (a) *ontology* – covering the nature of our being in the social world; (b) *stratification and emergence* – delineating the different, yet interlinked, domains of existence; (c) *epistemology* – addressing what we can know about the social world; (d) *ethics* – looking at the moral principles underpinning critical realism; and (e) *causality and change* – describing the theory of the dialectic lying at the heart of critical realism.

Ontology

For Bhaskar, actors shape their social worlds but are, in turn, constrained by social structures embedded in the fabric of social life. However, it is the nature of these structures that takes on a particular purchase in critical realism. In order to grasp the significance of social structure in critical realist philosophising, we must turn to Bhaskar's view of the social world. His ontological conceptualisation comprises three levels of reality, namely: (a) the *empirical* level, (b) the *actual* level and (c) the *causal* level. The first level is reflected in what we experience through our senses. We hear discordant themes in a piece of classical music eventually leading to a climax of resolution. We see a broad vista appear before us out of the mist. We taste a much anticipated, fortifying meal. These examples are of empirical engagement with reality through the senses.

In contrast, the actual level of reality is what happens regardless of our engagement with it. Hence, events occur beyond one's sensory experience. The fact that a person cannot hear a concert taking place in a faraway location does not mean that it has not occurred. One's range of sensory experience is truncated and restricted by spatial and temporal contexts yet there is still an awareness that others are 'going about their business' and life continues in 'faraway fields'. Reality does not have to be experienced by everyone for it to have ontological substance.

Last, the causal level has a major import in social life. Operating below the meniscus of the empirical and actual levels are unseen, causal mechanisms including many of the mechanisms generating adversity and trauma in people's lives. These mechanisms work synergistically to produce discernable effects in the empirical and actual levels of experience. In fact, by noting these effects we can hypothesise about the existence and nature of these mechanisms.

An example from the natural sciences illustrates this point. Thus, consider a sheet of paper splattered with iron filings. To the eye, there is nothing in the presentation of the filings signifying order. They appear as a random spread across the sheet. However, when a magnet is applied below the paper, the filings fall into a pattern around each pole of the magnet. The pattern is seen by the observer. It registers at the empirical level of reality. However, what is unseen is the mechanism of magnetism operating at the causal dimension. It is axiomatic that just because we cannot see immaterial forces with the naked eye, it does not mean they do not exist. Evolution has been an inexorable, causal mechanism in the phylogeny of human development yet has no visible properties *per se.*

These afore-mentioned examples come from the natural sciences. Yet, Bhaskar is keen to extend his thesis on the causal level to the psychological and social aspects of being. A second example from the psychological domain illustrates his stance with reference to the subject of childhood well-being. Take a young child removed from his parents' care and placed with a stranger. Most children who are securely bonded with their parents will show evident distress, anxiety and, ostensibly, rage given this situation. If the child is re-united with his parents after a short while, though, he slowly returns to his secure mode of being, feeling safe to explore and welcoming the parents' proximity. What the observer sees is the child's distress and subsequent calm. What is less clear, at this empirical level of observation, is what is causing the child's reaction when separating from, and reuniting with, his loving carers. In this regard, John Bowlby (2005), a child ethologist, suggested that children develop through an unseen mechanism of *attachment.* When they feel secure in their parents' care, they are empowered to explore their worlds and develop cognitive and social skills. However, when threatened, they return to their secure base.

Bowlby's work highlighted the existence of the psychosocial mechanism of attachment in social life. Beyond this domain, however, are wider social structural mechanisms operating at the causal level to make events happen, some of which lead to adverse consequences, others to fortuitous events. In neoliberal economies, for example, the pervasive mechanism of *commodification* acts to reduce social life to objects that have monetary value, that can be purchased, traded or cashed in. Commodification works in tandem with other neoliberal mechanisms such as deregulation, liberalisation and privatisation to shape the nature of modern life, its cultural forms, media representations and civic engagements. Empirical evidence (Wilkinson & Pickett, 2011) of growing inequalities, social pathologies and diminishing measures of well-being in many countries falling prey to the neoliberal global order testifies to the work of these unseen mechanisms operating within the sphere of political economy.

The combined effects of these mechanisms operating at the causal level create an unpredictable *smorgasbord* of cause and effect, with some mechanisms complementing each other, while others are acting in countervailing opposition. That said, far from being a deterministic philosophy, critical realism gives a central place to human agency in shaping outcomes in social life. Actors are affected by myriad mechanisms but, through their intentions in different times and social contexts, they often modify their effects. Therefore, causality is a complex affair involving the human being's subjective engagement with unseen forces that have an objective power.

Stratification and emergence

Such mechanisms operate within a stratified world comprising numerous, inter-lacing systems. In short, reality is layered. If the scientist targets one level of reality and identifies the mechanisms within it then, unquestioningly, there is an aspect of reality lying beneath it, one giving rise to its fundamental laws and processes. Thus, the characteristics of many animals and plants can be explained by physiological mechanisms but they, in turn, can be explained by deeper-level chemical mechanisms, a prominent one being photosynthesis. So, one can delve deeper, or 'drill down', increasingly into the microstructure of nano-particles.

Equally, reality builds from these microscopic layers to the larger social domains comprising institutions and political economy. This multilayered world can be studied by discrete disciplines ranging from quantum physics upward through physical chemistry, organic chemistry, physiology, psychology, the social sciences, humanities, philosophy and theology. In all of this, one layer of reality generates the next in a process of continual emergence yet, crucially, critical real-ism avoids attempts to reduce one layer to its deeper emergent base. For instance, human psychology should not be reduced to human biology and it to chemistry. Reductionist explanations fail to do justice to the discrete objective properties of each layer *sui generis*.

Epistemology

Bhaskar's articulation of the three different types of reality – empirical, actual and causal – constitutes the main frame of his ontology of the person-in-society. How-ever, what can be said regarding his view of epistemology? Here, Bhaskar makes a distinction between the *intransitive* and *transitive* dimensions. The former is the world that objectively exists. The latter is a human construction of that reality. In the transitive world, actors see reality through their perspectival lenses coloured as they may be by theory, bias, past experience and cultural habitus. This notion reverberates with Immanuel Kant's distinction between 'things-in-themselves' (the noumenal world) and 'things-as-we-see-them' (the phenomenal world), and our limited apprehension of the former through innate, *a priori* mental structures. Yet, as our theories develop over time, as social science evolves, the gap between the intransitive and transitive domains narrows, it is contended, much as in the metaphor of Plato's cave when light illuminates previously distorted and misap-prehended images revealing a more perspicacious view of reality as it really is.

Ethics

These central tenets on the nature of ontology and epistemology are comple-mented by a discerned position on ethics. In this context, critical realism does not subscribe to the notion of a value-free science which maintains 'the facts – value' distinction defended rigorously by many positivists. Critically, if one discovers the presence of oppressive mechanisms operating at the causal level of reality, then the social scientist is morally obligated to apply measures to negate their effects or at least expose them for what they are. Hence, when discovering the alienating effects of commodification, one might advocate for de-commodifying measures (for example, removing means-testing procedures from welfare entitlements). In this way, Bhaskar sees a connection between the production of knowledge in society and human emancipation. Essentially, negative value judgements can be made on phenomena which can be shown, through reason, argument or evidence, to be false, hegemonic, misanthropic or exploitative. There must be a presumption in favour of making the truth of the case known through what we have found in our research endeavours.

Causality and change

Bhaskar went on to further develop his thinking on causality and change in his path-breaking work, *Dialectic: The Pulse of Freedom* (1993). Here, he presented an in-depth examination of the *dialectic* as a force for transformation, freedom and emancipation: three imbricated areas that are central to critical social work practice. In order to make this case, Bhaskar critiqued (what he saw as) Hegel's misplaced view of the dialectic. When considering change, Hegel had made the mistake of starting affirmatively with what was present (that is, 'identity'). He then proceeded to consider how this presence was overcome, negated and subsumed through the contradictions it generated in a dynamic movement toward the whole. Over time, according to Hegel, the dialectical impulse would transcend contradiction and act as a progressive, cumulative movement toward a final totality.

By way of contrast, Bhaskar argued that dialectical processes did not necessarily eventuate in synthesis, nor were they determined by an unfolding positive teleology, or characterised by opposition. Rather, such forces might be signified by connection, separation or juxtaposition. Stating this another way, the dialectic could be regarded as any interplay between differentiated but related causal elements. Causal powers were a mix of interconnection as much as distinction. Overall, Bhaskar attempted to unravel the dialectic from its Hegelian moorings.

So, rather than starting with 'identity', (that is, what was there, or present), as Hegel had done, Bhaskar contended strongly that 'absence', (that is, what was not present), was the defining, inexorable starting point or prime mover of the dialectical impulse. 'Absence' was the *sine qua non* of change: the impetus for the removal or 'absenting' of constraints on human flourishing. To be clearer, 'absence' was synonymous with 'non-being', 'non-existence' or 'negation'. It could refer to a deficit in our conscious thinking (for example, our lack of awareness or understanding of the role of hegemonic powers in social life), or an absence of some entity, property or attribute (for instance, an impecunious existence marked by the social ills of poverty and isolation). Critically, 'absence' was ontologically real, concrete and tangible as opposed to existing at the level of mere ideation (as Hegel would have it).

The notion of something being 'absent', conceived of as a noun, could be thought of etymologically in another way, argued Bhaskar. Thus, the corollary of the noun was the verb 'to absent'. Simply put, 'to absent' meant to remove some lack or deficit. We might attempt, as social workers, to eliminate or 'absent' constraining social forces, perhaps xenophobia, that lead to stigmatisation and shame. Alternatively, the absenting focus might be on patriarchy, racism or sectarianism. This is the 'absenting' of 'absence': the eradication of something, or a property or state of affairs that has deleterious consequences for social well-being. Expressed somewhat differently, social justice eventuates out of incompleteness.

'Absenting' could also be subversive and iconoclastic and result in conscientisation: a position where the contradictions in life are understood and acted on. A conscious, critical awareness of 'absence', and the conjoined process of 'absenting', was the lynchpin of the dialectic, argued Bhaskar. 'Absenting' absence is consequently a driving negativity, a negativity that propels change. 'Negativity is the hub not only of existence but also of causality. Quite simply, to cause is to absent' (1993, p. 240). Out of insuperable incompleteness, or 'absence', arise various types of contradiction, dissonance, bind, strain, tension and discord that inject a yearning for freedom in subaltern populations. These contradictions come to the fore when human needs are not being met, or are being threatened. Clearly, absences have causal effects: a government moves to pump prime austerity measures culminating in a legitimation crisis that forces a political climb down; the absence of social support following a bereavement causes depression in a vulnerable subject. Not having something can generate the agitation preceding change, the restlessness of activism.

Bhaskar's arguments for the analytical primacy of 'absence' (over 'presence') in propelling social justice have merit. To apprehend any entity, we must be aware of what it is not – its 'absence'. Any kind of identification of an object presumes that we are aware of the conjoined state where the object does not exist. Thus, a conception of material well-being is underpinned by the related notion of penury and vice versa. In this way, 'absence' and 'presence' exist in a conceptual bipolarity that is ingrained in human thought. Moreover, it seems fallacious to view change as coming from 'presence': social change arises when the human subject is aware of what he or she lacks. Human rights are predicated on infringements, past status injustices, reification, or the objectification of the person (Nussbaum, 1995). Recognition eventuates out of misrecognition (Honneth, 1995).

Arguably, social work is a profession that ought to be critically attuned to 'absence' in the psychological domain of broken narrative, trauma, loss and attachment but also on the societal plane of marginalisation, exclusion, deprivation, incarceration and dispossession. Vitally, what critical realism offers to social work is an understanding of the deep-rooted, unseen (to the empirical eye) causal mechanisms that engender and sustain such absences and also the ones that lead to the absenting of such absences. Critical realism empowers social workers to 'drill down' below the meniscus of the everyday empirical world as part of an inquiry into 'depth' rather than skimming superficially on the plane of 'surface' impression.

With 'absence' at the heart of the transformative process, we can now consider Bhaskar's overarching view of the dialectic, comprising four critical moments, namely: *non-identity, negativity, totality* and *transformative praxis*. It is best to describe these interlinked moments though a practical example. A perilous food shortage in a country becomes apparent and we need to analyse the situation to arrive at credible solutions and change strategies to address the problem. The first moment of *non-identity* involves an analysis of some of the causal, generative mechanisms operating at the 'real' level of reality which might include natural, environmental factors (for example, drought, pestilence, water shortages or the effects of pollution). Here, we are factoring in the awareness that reality is stratified, differentiated and emergent, and therefore that the problem must be investigated at these different levels. What Bhaskar means, essentially, is that we must not be led down a blind alley of only looking at the problem though the lens of the 'empirical': what our sense impressions make of the problem. We may see things and hear things but they are only occluded impressions.

The second moment, *negativity*, looks critically at what is 'absent' in the situation and how to transform that absence through working with the contradictions it generates. Absence in the example proffered might refer to the loss of health, adequate nutrition, the right to life and social well-being. It could highlight contradictions in governmental policies aimed at resourcing local communities in times of need, create oppositional movements, in terms of local activism, and lead to advocacy at the internal level of aid.

The third moment, of *totality*, considers how events are caused by a raft of interconnected processes operating at the 'micro', 'mezzo' and 'macro' levels of reality. In the example posited, we could consider how psychological, social, environmental, economic, political and cultural mechanisms, operating at the level of the 'real', create and sustain the food shortage. For instance, neoliberal policies of free trade, austerity, circumscribed aid and unregulated markets might provide an important backdrop to the reluctance to intervene politically in the issue. The notion of totality requires us to think ecologically and in a systemic way about causation, taking account of how various contingencies operate in an imbricated way to affect people, social groupings, institutions and societies. Totality rests on the premise that phenomena must be seen as part of the whole and, that while the former is determined by the latter, both are equiprimordial.

The last moment, *transformative praxis*, occurs when we combine our analysis resulting from the previous three steps. Based on this holistic constellation, we are now in a position to understand more fully the deep-rooted causes of the problem, not on a surface, superficial level but in terms of the domain of the 'real'. Actors can reflect on this deeper understanding and initiate transformative measures to attain desired goals. Thus, an international aid agency can develop and institute a perspicacious change strategy aimed at enhancing positive generative mechanisms while ameliorating the negative ones.

Problem-based learning and critical realism

Problem-based learning (Clouston et al., 2010) is an educational method which involves students in formulating a problem in the classroom, and then supports them to examine it systematically as active learners. We can trace its origins back to Socratic forms of critical inquiry and Aristotelian attempts to interrogate 'appearances' so that our understanding of them deepens. A more recent philosopher, Dewey (1944), also embraced the essence of the approach by arguing that knowledge-acquisition was an active process, one involving a problem-solving course of development. The role of the educator was therefore to:

> organize education so that natural active tendencies shall be fully enlisted in doing something, while seeing to it that the doing requires observation, the acquisition of information, and the use of a constructive imagination, is what needs to be done to improve social conditions.
>
> (p. 137)

There are a number of central principles underpinning the problem-based learning stance, namely that:

- Learning is an active and developmental process shaped by a range of psychosocial, contextual factors such as past experience, achievement, access to learning resources and method of instruction;
- Students are active learners who bring their experiences and perspectives to create meaning when faced with challenging scenarios in the classroom;
- Educators are viewed as 'facilitators', 'cognitive coaches' or 'pedagogic mentors', as opposed to formal 'chalk and talk disseminators', of knowledge;
- The learning experience revolves around the consideration of a relevant, open-ended problem that serves as a catalyst or stimulus for critical inquiry;
- Knowledge-acquisition is student-centred and occurs within small groups who take ownership of the problem-solving process by applying relevant knowledge, recommended resources and past learning;
- Active learning involves applying, not only relevant domain knowledge but also critical thinking skills, so that students become effective problem-solvers;
- The educator, as facilitator, guides exploration, and stimulates critical thinking, reflection, problem-solving and reflexivity, by providing a theoretical scaffold for inquiry, understanding, knowledge-acquisition and learning;
- The problem under inquiry is 'open-ended' requiring students to embrace notions of complexity, fluidity, inter-connectedness, contradiction and spatio-temporal contingency; and
- Students are encouraged to form and test hypotheses concerning the underlying mechanisms ostensibly causing and ameliorating the problem.

These principles, which can be viewed as essentially constructivist in orientation, inform a typical problem-based learning process of inquiry. This starts with an elicitation of the problem. Essentially, students should feel that the problem resonates with their core interests, needs, tasks and responsibilities. It must be worth the attention. If the subject matter is nugatory, it will be hard to sustain their interest. Problem identification is therefore a process of mutual deliberation and often driven by ethical considerations or unresolved exigencies within the practice field.

The next step involves the facilitator guiding the students to a procedure or scaffold for investigating the problem. This helps to provide direction when it comes to examining the problem and brainstorming ways of addressing it. In other words, it generates practical advice on how to think through the problem systematically, analytically and thoroughly. As Gallagher (1997, p. 337) says, 'students receive systematic instruction in conceptual, strategic, and reflective reasoning in the context of a discipline that will ultimately make them more successful in later investigations'. For example, the process at this stage might involve setting out initial premises about the problem, followed by any facts that can be gathered about it, any theoretical considerations relating to it, the learning implications coming from these deliberations, and finally an action plan for resolving it. Later on, I will argue that the critical realist, investigative process, known as retroduction, fulfils this role amply.

After the above step has been clarified, it is a matter of enacting it, preferably in small sub-groups (of four to five students). Critically, the students must take responsibility for this step of inquiry using the facilitator as a resource person. The facilitator can direct the students to useful conceptual frameworks or theories that might illuminate different dimensions of the problem but these domains of knowledge are not exclusive or exhaustive. Students at this stage are encouraged to think laterally, logically, experimentally and hypothetically. They are also asked to think reflexively by examining how their assumptions about the problem reflect their own personal and social characteristics. Essentially, how does their class, race, age, gender and culture influence their construction of the problem?

As soon as each of the sub-groups has completed their inquiries into the problem, they are invited to reassemble into the large group. Here, each sub-group reports on their findings including their analysis of the problem and action plan for resolving it. Participants are encouraged to share any evidence for their conclusions, how they have applied critical thinking and made use of the theoretical scaffolding. Ideas and facts are shared. Key learning issues are highlighted. Any additional learning resources are indicated. Importantly, any new information is proffered.

When each group has reported on these areas, the facilitator helps the participants to evince summative themes and learning points, both on the causation of the problem, and also on the means for tackling it. Any disagreements on problem causation are debated. The facilitator will try to work toward a consensual understanding within the large group based on reasoned argumentation and evidence. The force of better argument should prevail.

Finally, the participants are asked to evaluate their own performance, their subgroup's contribution and that of the whole group. Essentially, how effective have they been in connecting with the problem, generating ideas and hypotheses about it, searching for facts and analysing feelings, formulating learning issues and developing a plan of action? Moreover, to what extent did they probe sufficiently, adopt higher-level thinking, utilise reflection and, critically, use group processes in a positive, collegiate way?

Clearly, there is a deep affinity between these learning principles and processes, and the critical realist precepts outlined earlier on. First, the emphasis on the student as an active inquirer, or co-producer of knowledge and action, chimes with critical realism's view of the human subject as possessing transformative agency. Thus, even though there are wider structural constraints inhibiting and reproducing knowledge-manufacture and action, people can make virtuosic responses, bringing individual interpretation and meaning to socially construct their social worlds. To reiterate, Bhaskar's final moment in his articulation of the dialectic is the appreciation of the transformative praxis that arises from reflexive awareness of 'absence' in social life.

Second, the focus on a deep-seated exploration of an open-ended problem, where learners appreciate the reality of complex and multifaceted causality, reverberates strongly with the critical realist emphasis on the 'real' domain of cause and effect, the domain that goes beyond the 'empirical' level of seen and felt experience. Problem-based learning, furthermore, acknowledges that reality comprises imbricated, intermeshed, internal and external causal processes much like Bhaskar's notion of 'totality' where an understanding of absence necessitates a comprehension of how subsystems affect the whole system and how the whole system, in turn, shapes the subsystems.

Third, the need for a method, or procedure of inquiry, within problem-based learning (as set out above) can be compared with critical realism's advocacy of *retroduction* as an analytical process for gaining insight into causation. The next section will explore this process in some detail as, within critical realism, it is the problem-solving method *par excellence*. The contention, here, is that it can be introduced to students within the problem-solving sequence explained earlier. Thus, the argument is that retroduction becomes the principal tool of inquiry within problem-based learning and that the critical realist ideas outlined earlier act as a theoretical source supporting the problem-solving process.

Retroduction, dialectical change and problem-based learning

Sayer (1992) says retroduction involves the inference from a description of some phenomena or problem to an understanding of the causal properties producing it. In retroduction, the researcher seeks to apprehend how an event 'B', the problem, was produced by 'A'. This is an *a priori* process of thinking backward, one that tries to identify the causal mechanisms giving rise to the event. To expand on the nature of this investigation, the inquirer starts with a *transcendental* question. Kant said such questions should take the following form: 'what must be the case in order for events to occur as they do'? In other words, an inquirer has observed something of interest – in this case, the problem – and now wants to understand the factors that have brought it about.

Inquirers respond to transcendental questions by developing hypotheses about what causal mechanisms may be operating in a given sphere. Such hypotheses often take the form of metaphorical hunches, inferences, models or analogies rather than tightly defined, scientific conjectures that are meant to be tested empirically in controlled conditions. For example, a study of the properties of electrons might compare them to the flow of water molecules along a river. Alternatively, a study of organisational life might compare it to a psychic prison. On the other hand, a study of patients in a mental hospital might conjecture that the experience amounts to a divestiture of their social identities. In retroduction, the aim is to hypothesise about the likely influence of multiple mechanisms producing interlinked effects on social life.

Given this complex task, the inquirer needs to draw on theories that purport to examine deep, causal properties in psychological and social life to gain a tentative understanding of what mechanisms are at play. For example, in social research, these may be theories of identity, face-to-face interaction and institutional life. Additionally, retroduction can be linked with *complexity theory* (Mason, 2008): the construction of an overall system by defining its constituent parts (or subsystems) and how they are linked together to produce discernable effects.

Once hypothetical mechanisms have been elicited, the inquirer then seeks for evidence to either confirm or disconfirm their presence. For example, if a mechanism of commodification were really at work, then the inquirer would expect to see evidence of human life being reduced to monetary factors or life being intractably linked to market principles. If, however, evidence from the empirical world is lacking, then alternative hypotheses need to be propounded and tested (using perhaps a different set of theories), up until the point the inquirer has sufficient evidence to make a compelling case regarding some of the factors affecting causality in the area of inquiry pursued. This can compare with a medical physician who observes outward symptoms in the patient, develops hypotheses about their underlying causes, tests whether they are present and re-formulates her hypothesis if required.

Finally, if there is a strong case for believing that a number of oppressive mechanisms have been located, then the inquirer is duty bound to take actions to offset their effects. For example, if commodification is evidenced, the inquirer might resort to a set of policy recommendations highlighting the need for de-commodifying measures. In a welfare context, this could include arguments for removing means-testing for essential child-care services. In all of this, it is essential to remember that outcomes in social life are the combined effect of not only deep-seated mechanisms but also human agency working in specific temporal and spatial contexts. Human agents, far from being cultural dopes, reflect on their circumstances. They use conceptual space to deliberate on constraints and enabling factors and take action accordingly.

From what has been said, retroduction focuses on an event, or a problem to be understood, at a deep causal level. However, the notion of a problem-situation can be recast as an 'absence' to be interrogated, if we are to embrace Bhaskar's work on dialectical change. In other words, we start with a notion of 'absence' in social work: the lack of emotional well-being, the want for better housing conditions, the nonexistence of social amenities in a deprived area. What causes each of these absences and how do we *absent* them? To reiterate, the problem becomes synonymous with a defined 'absence'. This notion of an 'absence' kick-starts the retroductive, problem-solving process and its ensuing steps. So, the transcendental question asks: 'what must be the case for this particular 'absence' to exist as it does'? Secondly, 'how do we *absent* that absence'?

Retroduction, reworked in this way to accommodate the notion of 'absence' as the central driving force of inquiry, can be integrated within the problem-based learning approach, to enhance its capacity to unravel complex problems or absences. But how exactly? Earlier, it was suggested that problem-based learning relied on a procedure or scaffolding: a sequence of stages through which students might begin to examine the problem systematically. It is here that retroduction can be introduced and explained to social work students and examples provided showing its application to real-life situations of concern.

The challenge for social work education

Clearly, there are a set of conceptual and practical challenges for social work educators in integrating these separate, although compatible, elements of inquiry. First, there is the need to explain the essential tenets of critical realism and retroduction to students. Second, there is the necessity for students to understand the logistics of problem-based learning, its rationale, focus, steps and stages. Last, there is the challenge of integrating critical realism with the problem-based learning approach and enabling students to apply it to a chosen problem/absence. To take stock of these challenges, I suggest social work educators might consider structuring their input to students around three inter-linked orientations followed by a problem-based learning project. At the outset, these dimensions of the learning input should be briefly summarised before addressing them in more detail. At this beginning stage, it is important that students realise the value of combining an active, student-centred learning approach with a philosophical perspective aimed at understanding human oppression.

The first orientation aims to present the core tenets of critical realism (covered earlier) to the students, including the retroductive inquiry process. Because critical realism is largely theoretical and conceptual in content, and hence does not lend itself to easy explanation, it is important to provide examples from the social world demonstrating its applicability. I have provided some illustrations in this chapter. In addition, students should be encouraged to read the existing social work literature on critical realism, most of which I have summarised or referenced earlier. Primarily, this first orientation seeks to enable students to move from 'surface' to 'depth', to inquire below the meniscus of everyday sense impressions. Practical examples can help, but educators might also resort to metaphors to clarify key concepts. For example, the notion of stratification might be represented analogously with reference to the structure of a Russian doll with its nested figurines.

The second orientation involves explaining the problem-based learning approach to students. The principles and processes underpinning it, described earlier, could be clarified by providing examples of how it might be used to tackle a problem in social work that students may have encountered while on placement. How to marry the need for relationship-based social work with the demands of organisational regulation is perhaps a common challenge within Anglophile countries. Thus, the model is presented both conceptually but is also anchored within real-life demands. The educator should remind students that they will get a further opportunity to understand the model by applying it later on to a problem/absence of their choice.

The third orientation attempts to meld, or merge, critical realist thinking within the problem-based learning method. I have suggested that this is best done by introducing critical realism as an overarching theoretical scaffolding for analysing the chosen problem/absence. In doing so, students are encouraged to view the problem through a realist lens: one which involves an inquiry into depth, and the unseen causal mechanism perpetuating and assuaging the problem. Importantly, the retroductive process allows students, acting as self-directed learners, to draw on a wide range of theories to explain what is happening beneath the surface. Human behaviour in social work can be understood, *inter-alia*, through attachment and object-relations theories, social learning theory, systemic perspectives, and through bio-psycho-social understandings of the person in her environment (Pilgrim, 2015). Critical realism requires students to construct hypotheses about the problem/absence by using pertinent theories. More than that, it requires them to test the plausibility of the hypothesis. Without question, they are active learners in this process.

The final stage of learning invites students to apply the third orientation to a problem in social work of their choice. This is the practical component of the learning sequence and can be viewed as a working project. It is meant to broadly apply the stages of the problem-based learning method (outlined earlier) albeit using retroduction as the prototypical, problem-solving procedure. This will necessitate students working in small groups as advocated by the method, reporting back to the larger group on their findings, with the social work facilitator/educator drawing out summative learning themes at the end of the process. It is vital at this stage of practical implementation that social work educators reiterate the meaning of complex ideas (as and when needed), and remind students of the process being followed, acting as an informational resource when there is confusion or when students are veering off the task.

Conclusion

So, to summarise, I am suggesting that critical realism offers social work students a veritable way of thinking about the social world in order to understand the deep-seated causes of different events, including critical absences in social life. Because it has mostly been articulated as an abstract body of thought, it presents challenges for the social work educator when applying it to real-life situations.

Social work educators, it is contended, can rise to this challenge, by integrating critical realist ideas and procedures within the problem-based learning approach. Because the latter focuses on real-life problems, or absences to be solved, it acts as a vehicle for critical realist problem-solving in social work. Not only do both approaches share a similar approach to human agency, the need for transformative praxis, and the nature of problem formation and causation, they also insist on a robust means of interrogating problems to elicit causative factors and to plan action strategies. Centrally, both start with a problem or absence to be determined. In short, they are commensurate and compatible sources of understanding.

More specifically, by co-opting the retroductive procedure within the problem-based learning sequence of inquiry, students move from a surface exploration of the problem/absence to one of depth understanding. Additionally, they are given a practical *modus operandi* for utilising critical realist ideas which, arguably, should be linked to real-world concerns, if they are to have any meaning at all. Problem-based learning provides a lens through which critical realism can be viewed in a practical way, as it grounds the approach, making it relevant to social work concerns. *Ipso facto*, critical realism invigorates problem-based learning and it, in turn, widens the accessibility and applicability of critical realism: the connection is symbiotic. Viewing this another way, social work students need to see the relevance of ideas for practice. Problem-based learning provides this template of understanding, and it is one that social work educators, who are animated by critical realist ideas, might consider using.

References

Bhaskar, R. (1978) *A Realist Theory of Science*, Brighton: Harvester Press.
Bhaskar, R. (1993) *Dialectic: The Pulse of Freedom*, London: Verso.
Bhaskar, R. (1998) *The Possibility of Naturalism: A Philosophical Critique of the Contemporary Human Sciences*, London: Routledge.
Blom, B., & Moren, S. (2010) Explaining social work practice – The CAIMeR theory, *Journal of Social Work*, 10(1), 98–119.
Bowlby, J. (2005) *The Making and Breaking of Affectional Bonds*, London: Routledge.
Briar-Lawson, K. (2012) Critical realism: Response to Longhofer and Floersch, *Research on Social Work Practice*, 22(5), 523–528.
Clouston, T., Wescott, L., Whitcombe, S., Riley, J., & Matheson, R. (2010) *Problem-Based Learning in Health and Social Care*, London: Wiley-Blackwell.
Craig, D., & Bigby, C. (2015) Critical realism in social work research: Examining participation of people with intellectual disability, *Australian Social Work*, 68(3), 309–323.
Dewey, J. (1944) *Democracy and Education*, New York: The Free Press.
Gallagher, S. (1997) Problem-based learning: Where did it come from, what does it do, and where is it going? *Journal for the Education of the Gifted*, 20(4), 332–362.
Honneth, A. (1995) *The Struggle for Recognition: The Moral Grammar of Social Conflicts*, Cambridge, MA: MIT Press.
Houston, S. (2005) Philosophy, theory and method in social work: Challenging empiricism's claim on evidence-based practice, *Journal of Social Work*, 5, 7–20.
Houston, S. (2010) Prising open the black box: Critical realism, action research and social work, *Qualitative Social Work*, 9(1), 73–91.

Houston, S. (2012) Reviewing the coming crisis in social work: A response to Lonhofer and Floersch, *Research on Social Work Practice*, 22, 520–522.

Knowles, M., Holton, E., & Swanson, R. (2005) *The Adult Learner*, London: Elsevier.

Locke, J. (1700/1979) *An Essay Concerning Human Understanding*, Oxford: Clarendon Press.

Longhofer, J., & Floersch, J. (2012) The coming crisis in social work: Some thoughts on social work and science, *Research on Social Work Practice*, 22(5), 520–522.

Longhofer, J., & Floersch, J. (2014) Values in a science of social work: Values-informed research and research-informed values, *Research on Social Work Practice*, 24(5), 527–534.

Mäntysaari, M. (2005) Realism as a foundation for social work knowledge, *Qualitative Social Work*, 4(1), 87–98.

Mason, M. (2008) *Complexity Theory and the Philosophy of Education*, Chichester: Wiley-Blackwell.

Nussbaum, M. (1995) Objectification, *Philosophy and Public Affairs*, 24(4), 249–291.

Oliver, C. (2012) Critical realist grounded theory: A new approach, *British Journal of Social Work*, 42(2), 371–387.

Pilgrim, D. (2015) *Understanding Mental Health: A Critical Realist Exploration*, London: Routledge.

Sayer, A. (1992) *Method in Social Science: A Realist Approach*, London: Routledge.

Part III

6 Understanding the dynamics between professional social and welfare work and social politics

A critical realist perspective

Monica Kjørstad

Introduction

The aim of this article is to discuss how a critical realist approach can be used as an analytical tool to understand the dynamics of the relationship between social politics, institutions of social welfare and professional social and welfare implementation work. To illustrate the discussion, I will use an empirical project about social workers' implementation of a workfare policy in Norway, as an example. The project attempted to describe and analyze the dialectic relation between over-arching institutional relationships such as the body of laws and existing policies, institutional practices and the practice of social workers. A central issue was to investigate challenges and ethical dilemmas confronting professional social workers who were responsible for the implementation of a workfare policy in Norway (Kjørstad, 2008c; 2016 a [2005]).

In the first part of the article, I will present my theoretical and methodological considerations and reflections. Then follows a description of the project and an illustration of how I understand a typical *Context – Mechanism – Outcome* (C-M-O) configuration as a design for the project (Pawson & Tilley, 1997). Finally, I will discuss the relevance and potential of critical realism as an ontology for understanding the complex dynamics in a field of practice. This will also demonstrate the interplay between the accumulation of knowledge in practical day-to-day work and the theoretical deliberation of abstractions.

The concrete field of action: theoretical and analytical perspectives

Social science phenomena are characterised by complexity, by their dependence on context and by the interplay among several motivating forces. This involves theoretical and methodological challenges for the study of implementation practices and their consequences. For knowledge to be applicable, we must first assume that we are acquainted with the mechanisms that produce empirical events, even if they not are directly observable. This implies that pure empiricism has limited value in the explanation of human action (Bhaskar, 1978; Sayer, 2008).

In the project, I chose to describe critical realism by contrasting it to empirical realism. Critical realism emphasises the search for fundamental relationships and mechanisms which constitute the phenomenon under study and this distinguishes it from empiricism. Both empiricism and critical realism presuppose that reality exists independent of the observer, but in empiricism a second presupposition claims that knowledge of reality is directly in reach of the researcher on the basis of meticulous studies based on observation. In addition, empiricism attempts to reduce the importance of the observer's role and of contextual relationships. Research is directed toward finding empirical regularities that have the character of general laws. Empiricism contains an input-output perspective in relation to the phenomenon under study, which is viewed as being a 'black box'. A decisive difference in relation to critical realism is that critical realism is directed at opening the black box and uncovering the generative mechanisms that influence a specific outcome. Generative mechanisms are theoretical phenomena – i.e. abstractions that one may use as a starting point to clarify and interpret reality. The phenomena that research attempts to understand are often created by mechanisms operating at several levels of reality – i.e. reality is seen as being stratified (Danermark et al., 2002).

This understanding has been central for the selection of the design for this project. A critical discourse analytic approach was chosen, which made interpretation and reflection possible (Fairclough,1992; 1995). Critical discourse analysis distinguishes itself ontologically from various post-structural forms of discourse analysis (e.g. text analysis), in the sense that it includes *reality* as this is understood within a critical realist perspective – i.e. social and material relationships in society exist and are dialectically related to the actors that compose the societal system (Fairclough, 1995). In this perspective, discursive elements are dialectically related to other social dimensions.

A characteristic that distinguishes critical realism from other forms of realism is the view that reality is divided into three domains (Bhaskar, 1986; Danermark et al., 2002). First, there is *the empirical domain* that includes that which we can observe. Next, there is *the factual domain* or the events and phenomena which actually occur, but which are not always observable. Finally, there is *the real domain* that includes the structures, mechanisms and everything else that is independent of the researcher. By incorporating a critical realist perspective, it is possible to better uncover and understand the connections among these domains (Fairclough, 1995). A central assumption is that the phenomena that we are studying are *real*, but that they do not always disclose themselves manifestly.

The dynamic relation between society, institutions and professionals

When public programs are put into effect, we encounter a three-dimensional relationship among the state, the implementing party and the citizen (Rothstein,

2001; 1998). These three parties are following different logics and consequently they are subjected to different feedback mechanisms that sometimes might be a source of conflict. Problems of implementation are often described as being either a characteristic of the decision-makers or a characteristic of those who implement their decisions. Focusing on decision-makers, critics point to unclear goals, vague and ambiguous political resolutions, cases that are merely a matter of political symbolism or the lack of resources to fully implement plans. When welfare professionals who implement decisions are in focus, critics point to skepticism or opposition to political decisions because their professional judgment is not in sync with the policies they are expected to put into effect. Another reason for problems of implementation are the differences in opinion between upper-level executives in the organization and those who are at lower levels regarding the effects and utility of the political resolutions that are to be implemented (Sannerstedt, 2001). These are matters of importance for relationships between decision-makers and those who are expected to implement their decisions.

The traditional way of seeing the relationship between norms and societal institutions is that a solely institutional structure for social, political and economic relationships depends on cultural norms which are shared by members of society. However, the connections in this causal chain may be reversed. As fellow citizens, we decide to a considerable degree which social norms will be prevalent in society, because we can choose how we want to construct our political institutions (Rothstein, 1998). Politics, understood as being a conscious design of political institutions and political programs, cannot solely be explained by referring to the encompassing society. It has its own clarifying powers (Ibid.).

The discretion given to professionals

A great deal of the responsibility for implementing workfare, with considerable room for professional discretion, has been delegated to the public administrative system. This implies that normative and ethical research questions within bureaucracy are central. In this connection, it has been of special interest to analyze situations where the professional integrity of social workers has been challenged by the legal framework requiring that evaluations regarding the conditions for the provision of social assistance are made on a case-by-case basis. In these situations, it is particularly important that the social worker is attentive to the needs of clients to make their own decisions (Kjørstad, 2008a). This area has great importance for the individual claimant, but it can be unclear who has the responsibility for decisions: a kind of *no man's land in the welfare state* (Vike et al., 2002).

There are diverse ways in which matters of implementation are presented in the literature of political science. One perspective (the 'top-down' approach) argues that decision-makers determine political resolutions and the executives below them in the bureaucracy implement their decisions in a more or less mechanical way. The preconditions for this to be a functionally good description are that there are clear relationships between the goals of policy and the means to achieve those goals, and goals must be simple and not open to discussion. This perspective builds on a rationalistic view of implementation. An antithesis to this view has been presented by Michael Lipsky in his description of *grass-roots* bureaucrats (Lipsky, 1980). The perspective is used to describe professionals who work directly with people – for example, nurses, social workers and teachers. In such cases, he argues that relationships between goals and means are often unclear and goals are complex and open to discussion. Professional practitioners, in these cases, have been delegated the authority to make decisions and have a great deal of discretion in tackling their assignments. In reality, it is not politicians, but professionals who create policy in their fields of action and expertise. Their activities are based on the delegated authority to make decisions. In the encounter between a professional practitioner and a client, the professional is given the discretion to make decisions that are based on professional insight in order to take actions that are in the best interests of the client. In this way, professional practitioners form elements of public policy. The content of the work they do is determined by professional norms about legitimate knowledge in the cases before them. 'The sum total of their actions constitute the implementation of public policy in their field of action' (Rothstein, 2001). The degree to which their actions are in sync with resolutions taken in the political systems is an open question.

Ethical implications of workfare as a social policy

The concept of workfare has ideological power specifically because it is an imprecise and ambiguous concept. It may include rights and duties, coercion and care, exclusion and inclusion. The concrete solution to the problem of providing boundaries for the concept is characterised by which dimensions are given weight and depends on the general economic and ideological climate (Midré, 1995). Concepts that are often articulated in the rhetoric of the workfare discourse include *activation, participation, responsibility, rights and duties*. It is common to point out that the logic of contract and exchange has substantially influenced the thinking that grounds social policy development. More and more often, welfare benefits are seen as being *traded* for work.

In professional discourse, the question of the application of universal ethical rules as a guide for action is contested. The main argument against it is that the ethical and moral choices that professionals have to make is situation dependent and local. The other side points to the importance of a universal normative foundation for society. Universal rules are needed to guard against a breach of generally accepted norms, to secure basic rights, and to ensure the appropriate use of professional power.

A central question when considering the workfare policy from an ethical perspective, is whether society should allow people social benefits instead of income from working (supposing that there *is* work). This moral question gets its 'answer' in the social security law which states that everybody can apply for help for housing and living, and that this kind of help must be given in cooperation with the client. The autonomy of the client is strongly expressed in universal human rights and in the international ethical codex for social workers.

These questions raise some of the fundamental problems that are related to the role of professions in the welfare state. In the practical work in the public service institutions, the public servants have to make decisions based on professional judgement that are *in between* administrative rules and the autonomy of the service user (Kjørstad, 2008a; 2016a [2005]; 2016b). In this field, administrative discretion takes place. The professional social and welfare worker will constantly be confronted by these challenges, having a position 'between a rock and a hard place'.

The project

The research in Norway on the effects of workfare has primarily been directed at the outcome variable – i.e. the number of clients that gain employment after a goal-oriented activation program has been undertaken, or alternatively, the number of clients that have failed to find employment. Very little attention has been given to the internal processes in the institutions that carry out this policy. The concrete point of implementation, primarily the municipal social welfare office or the local labor office, is viewed as being a 'black box' (Latour, 1987; Latour, 2000; Morén & Blom, 2003). There is limited knowledge about the way in which the policy has been implemented in practice, and little or no clarifications that explain why results have or have not been achieved. On the other hand, several research projects have concluded that social welfare clients that have received social assistance because of their lack of employment have deeper and more extensive social problems and health problems than were previously known (Lødemel & Trickey, 2001). There seems to be a gap between the intentions and results of workfare as a social policy.

My intention with this project was to illuminate the norm-setting function of institutions in light of practical social work with implementing a workfare – or welfare to work – policy in the public services in Norway. The focus is on the way in which social workers *practice* workfare and the different strategies that are utilised in its implementation. A central assumption of this approach is the hypothesis that the implementation of workfare is a complicated interaction that incorporates many variables that can be difficult to disclose. It has been necessary to draw attention away from the social worker as an individual agent and focus on the societal, political and traditional ways of thinking that influence and constitute the room to maneuver that social workers can utilise. Practices at the micro-level and the internal discourses can contribute to make the implementation of a specific social policy visible, but they can also contribute to hide some aspects of the overarching policies and the intentions of the law. The field of practice can be seen as a creative field that has opportunities for change within it (Fairclough, 1992; 1995).

An intensive design

The project was a small-scale, qualitative study. A multidimensional approach was chosen, based on observations of consultation interviews with the social workers, group interviews with heads of social agencies, case discussions and dialogue conferences with participants, and document studies. All parts of the research process, except the document studies, were videotaped. The research process may be subdivided into two main stages: the first stage consisted of the observations and the interviews, and the second stage consisted of the group interviews, the case conferences and the dialogue conferences (Kjørstad, 2008b).

The study was based on two theoretical perspectives. In the first one, the municipal social welfare office is seen as a *gate-keeping institution*. One aspect of gate-keeping is universal. Every society must decide who is to benefit from social provision and who is to be denied that provision, whenever provisions are made available that are not intended to include every member of society (Midré, 1995). In Norway, social workers are the ones who are expected to make those decisions. This has been referred to as a *gate-keeping* function (Terum, 1996).

The second theoretical perspective is based on a conception of *bureaucratic ethics* where ethical action is crucial (Lundquist, 1988; 1992). This perspective is related to the gate-keeping functions of public institutions and applies to the social worker when he or she occupies a bureaucratic position. Social workers that are employed in bureaucratic organisations must relate to a number of relationships that have ethical potential: to clients, colleagues, employers, politicians and the public at large (Kjørstad, 2008c; 2016a/2005).

Figure 6.1 illustrates how the relationship between structure and context, mechanism and outcome, is adapted to the project in a C-M-O configuration (Pawson & Tilley, 1997). The arrow on the lower right shows that the relationship is also influenced by other mechanisms, or conditions which can increase, reduce or counteract the outcome (effect/event). The figure illustrates a complex situation that involves an understanding of causality that is radically different from the empirical view that causality is solely a matter of empirically observed regularities.

The context is the social welfare office as a gate-keeping institution, where social workers encounter clients and determine the kinds of help to be given and the conditions that have to be met by clients to receive that help. Workfare is more or less automatically required when social assistance is applied for. It constitutes an aspect of the social treatment that is practised. It consists of a forcefully applied filtering system in accord with the Norwegian law. Of course, the client's own preparedness, desires and motivations are also preconditions for the way in which the process unfolds.

At this level, one can uncover the forces and mechanisms that produce outcomes (Morén & Blom, 2003; Danermark et al., 2002). In this way, one is able to make the potential for change in social phenomena comprehensible, in addition to searching for structural causal factors. The effects of a generative mechanism are contextually conditioned – i.e. the context determines whether or not the mechanism is active, passive or if some other mechanism is at work to counter its effects

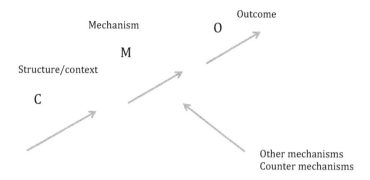

Figure 6.1 The C-M-O configuration

Source: Pawson and Tilley (1997); Sayer (2000).

(Pawson & Tilley, 1997). Actions mediate everyday social phenomena as well as deeper structural relationships that constitute the society under study.

Reciprocity as a generative mechanism

Several societal discourses that influence the development of professional practices are at work, both inside and outside the arena where the day-to day practices are unfolding. Common for many of the Western welfare states is an underlying fear of *welfare dependency* upon which the various reform programs promoting activation are based (Dahl & Lorentzen, 2003a; Dahl & Lorentzen, 2003b). Another argument that is used in the rhetoric surrounding workfare is the argument that workfare is a form of *rehabilitation*. In the *marginalisation* discourse, the argument is based on the idea that losing one's ties to the labor market will lead to exclusion and stigmatisation (Halvorsen, 1998).

The reciprocity discourse is perhaps the most challenging. In my examination of the way professional social workers carry out the workfare policy, I have interpreted the norm of reciprocity as one of the central mechanisms but also the least problematised societal norm. Reciprocity is a central element in the relationship between human beings. In general, it consists of the obligation to exchange goods or services on an equal basis. It can be seen as being a norm that contributes to holding society together (Gouldner, 1960; Kjørstad, 2016b).

Mutuality and reciprocity are based on the moral concepts of duty and obligation. Even though there is a widespread belief that reciprocity is important for holding society together, the concept is rather diffuse (Gouldner, 1960). Gouldner points out that the concept of reciprocity is "silently" involved and that differences in the degree of reciprocity are often denied. Although the norm ordinarily includes the duty to reciprocate only when the receiving individual has something he or she can use to repay the giver, this does not necessarily mean that there is any agreement about the receiver's ability to repay. For example, the norm is not applied in full strength in relationships to children and the elderly. One cannot require a moral obligation to repay from those who are poorly situated and who, at least periodically, do not have the possibility or ability to repay (Gouldner, 1960; White, 2000).

In my study, many of the professional social workers experienced an ethical dilemma in the presupposition that required them to demand that clients enter into a *contract* that is not reciprocal. The *principle of reciprocity*, in this case, refers to the idea that people should, in principle, give something back to society when they receive social benefits. From one ethical position, reciprocity presupposes *equality* between the parties involved in a contractual relationship. This becomes a problematic issue when clients who are desperately in need of housing, food and clothing are forced to agree to contracts that may limit or eliminate their only source of income.

Special kinds of mechanisms are institutionalised and leave their mark in every society – they function as so-called starting mechanisms for social interaction (Gouldner, 1960). Gouldner maintains that the norm of reciprocity is one such starting mechanism because the party that initiates gift-giving or service-rendering to another party can contribute to the establishment of a trusting relationship which makes further cooperation possible. It may be added that the very same act can also create a relationship of dependence. This may lead one to ask how the norm of reciprocity functions as a starting mechanism in the social work that is practised in public welfare administration.

Half a round of retroduction: observations from 'the outside' and experiences from 'the inside'

The data collected from the observations of the counselling of the clients and from the interviews with the social workers afterward were initially analysed. This gave a first impression of the challenges that social workers faced in their role as the front-line soldiers of social policy.

In the second stage, eight case conferences were held where the social work-ers in groups of four discussed which of their own cases that they considered *critical* (Fook, 2002), and felt they had not quite finished. Among the multitude of topics that were discussed, one issue turned out to be of central importance: the high degree of complexity of the life situations that were presented and the difficult task of working with these cases (Kjørstad, 2016b). In the discussion of the mechanisms at play, it became clear that the principle of reciprocity was dominating.

The relevance and potential of critical realism to study a field of practice: methodological considerations

The methodological approach is an example of an *intensive research design* that makes it possible to uncover generative mechanisms that work behind 'the observable' (Archer,2003; Bhaskar,2002; Danermark et al., 2002; Sayer, 2008).

Danermark et al. have called this attitude *critical methodological pluralism* argu-ing that the foundation for what is suitable or not is to be found in the relationship between metatheory and method (Archer et al., 1998; Danermark et al., 2002). This process may also be associated with a kind of 'hermeneutics of mutual curi-osity' that might avoid some of the adverse effects of 'hermeneutics of suspi-cion' (Ricoeur, 1981) that make practitioners feel uncomfortable and sometimes distrusted. The aim is that the researcher and the practitioner should develop mutual confidence and share a curiosity about the mechanisms that causes a specific practice to be successful or not, and how it may be corrected if that is necessary(Kjørstad, 2008b). This procedure is in accordance with the mandate that research in social work should take into consideration the consequences for those who are dependent on social assistance (Humphries, 2004).

The design for the project was constructed to handle qualitative data and does not necessarily accommodate society's demand for evidence-based research if this is defined as based on cause-and-effect explanations. If, however, evidence-based research is defined as based on assessment and interpretation, professional arguments and ethical deliberation, the project is an example of evidence-based research that may generate knowledge applicable for practice (Humphries, 2003).

Opening the 'black box'

The main bulk of research on public social services in Norway has been focused on problems where it has been appropriate to regard the social service office as a black box. The 'noise' from the rumble inside the box is often overlooked not to 'disturb' the research process. By reducing the content *inside* the box to input and output variables, a reduction of complexity is achieved. Depending on the context, this approach may have shortcomings (Kjørstad, 2008). In a critical real-ist perspective, it may represent an unduly simplification of reality; in this case what in fact is happening in the dialectic relation between structures and agency and between the actors (Archer, 2000; Archer et al., 1998; Bhaskar, 1986; 2002). To be able to get a better understanding of what was going on inside the box, we had to *open* it, observe what was going on, and try to understand the dynamics of social work practice from that position. The 'noise' that may be regarded as disturbance of the input-output process in a different research design was the very substance that we were searching for. During this process, 'raw data' were gradu-ally elaborated and transformed into practical knowledge. In this situation, facts and artefacts are created, maintained and changed within social processes (Latour, 1987). In combination with observations and interviews, the *articulating activi-ties* involved in case discussions and in the dialogue conferences have provided a more authentic picture of the implementation practice than one would have achieved from written texts alone (Floersch, 2000). The elaboration of everyday knowledge has opened up new research issues and stimulated the formulation of new research questions.

If one had chosen a black-box approach to measure the outcomes of implement-ing this social policy, one could have counted the number of clients that stopped applying for social assistance at social welfare offices with the passage of time. This might have provided useful knowledge, but it would not have explained what social workers were doing that either had positive or negative effects. I was interested in delving deeper – beyond 'the obvious'. By examining the project's different phases, by observing conversations with clients, by interviewing social workers and by carrying out dialogue conferences addressing theoretical perspectives, the picture I had of reciprocity as a generative mechanism gradually became clearer. What I found was that the norm of reciprocity thoroughly saturates the practice of social work, and that this may have negative consequences since it seldom suits the realities of the situation.

I wanted to involve social work practitioners in the interpretive process based on the assumption that the researchers and social work practitioners working together would be able to get a better grasp of reality. This implies that in practice the 'black box' could be opened. By opening up the research process to information, that in a typical input-output analysis would have been understood as *noise*, it became possible to get closer to reality.

Conclusion

In this project, I have examined the institutional and discursive practices at municipal social welfare agencies. By studying the practice of social workers and listen to their reflections on their own practices, I have attempted to gain an understanding of the generative mechanisms that are in play. *Reflection* is understood here as *ruminations concerning the presuppositions of their activities* and questioning what they have taken for granted (Alvesson & Deetz, 2000; Alvesson & Sköldberg, 2000). The research project has aimed at acquiring access to the practical insights and judgments of professional practitioners by discussing the researcher's interpretation of the data with those professional practitioners during the research process. By doing this, the validation of the data has been a continuing process (Kvale & Enerstvedt, 1995).

In my study, the norm of *reciprocity* was scrutinised. The norm of reciprocity is a concrete and special mechanism which creates motives for returning favors, even when power relationships invite one party to exploit the other. The present discourses in a policy field, for example discourses about social work within the field of unemployment, tell us something important about the structure of our institutions and their norm-setting and normative function in society. This is necessary if one wants to analyse a certain context to find underlying mechanisms that influence the implementation processes. This is what Stan Houston has formulated as *return to depth in practice* (Houston, 2001). Michel Foucault's genealogical project is much about doing so, but he never made any concrete theory out of it. Nevertheless, his discussions about uncovering *regimes of truth* is much about what critical realists have to do in their effort to finding underlying mechanisms behind the empirical surface (Deetz, 1988).

The methodology chosen has shown that it can be fruitful to explore an institution or a field of practice by using different approaches to capture a close picture of the context where the implementation of a policy is undertaken. This is done by utilising different methods and by studying the phenomena at several levels: societal, institutional and individual. Critical discourse analysis makes it possible to shed light upon the connection between the different levels (Fairclough, 1995). The approach begins by acknowledging that the phenomena under study are *real*, but that they are not always manifestly disclosed. The process can be compared with an archeological excavation, where researchers discover layer after layer in their findings. This is an analogue to critical realism's theory of stratification.

From that position, one may consider structural analysis and hermeneutics as complementary perspectives that refer to one another. As Paul Ricoeur stated: the structural analysis is *a step* – between surface interpretation and in-depth interpretation (Ricoeur, 1981). Ricoeur argues that it is possible to place clarification and interpretation within the same 'hermeneutic arch' and to integrate these two contradictory attitudes. *To clarify (or explain)* is to display the structure – i.e. the internal dependent relationships. Interpretation as appropriation occurs in the second part of the process.

The core purpose of professional social care and welfare work is to alleviate human misery. The critical realist perspective can contribute to this goal by enabling social workers to utilise deeper methods of inquiry and analysis to better understand and develop their profession. Its methodology presupposes that reality is stratified and that a many-layered understanding of reality is necessary. Critical realism looks for mechanisms at several levels. It is critically explorative and incites questions about matters that are ordinarily taken for granted. Normative research problems can be relevantly formulated and asked, including questions concerning justice in society. Critical realism has an interest in emancipation that can be used to shed light on the controversies regarding the causes and the effects of social exclusion.

References

Alvesson, M., & Deetz, S. (2000) *Kritisk samhällsvetenskaplig metod [Critical Social Science Methodology]*, Lund: Studentlitteratur.

Alvesson, M., & Sköldberg, K. (2000) *Reflexive Methodology: New Vistas for Qualitative Research*, London: Sage.

Archer, M. S. (2000) *Being Human: The Problem of Agency*, Cambridge: Cambridge University Press.

Archer, M. S. (2003) *Structure, Agency and the Internal Conversation*, Cambridge: Cambridge University Press.

Archer, M. S., Bhaskar, R., Collier, A., Lawson, T., & Norrie, A. (eds.) (1998) *Critical Realism: Essential Readings*, London: Routledge.

Bhaskar, R. (1978) *A Realist Theory of Science*, Sussex: Harvester Press.

Bhaskar, R. (1986) *Scientific Realism & Human Emancipation*, London: Verso.

Bhaskar, R. (2002) *Reflections on Meta-Reality: Transcendence, Emancipation and Everyday Life*, London: Sage.

Dahl, E., & Lorentzen, T. (2003a) Dynamics of social assistance: The Norwegian experience in comparative perspective, *International journal of Social Welfare*, 12, 289–301.

Dahl, E., & Lorentzen, T. (2003b) Explaining exit to work among social assistance recipients in Norway: Heterogeneity or dependency? *European Sociological Review*, 19, 519–536.

Danermark, B., Ekström, M., Jakobsen, L., & Karlsson, J. C. (2002) *Explaining Society: Critical Realism in the Social Sciences*, London: Routledge.

Deetz, S. (1988) Discursive Formations, Strategized Subordination and Self Surveillance. In McKinlay, A. & Starkey, K. (eds.), *Foucault, Management and Organization Theory*, London: Sage, pp. 151–172.

Fairclough, N. (1992) Critical discourse analyses and the marketization of public discourse: The universities, *Discourse and Society*, 4(2), 133–168.

Fairclough, N. (1995) *Critical Discourse Analysis*, London: Longman.

Floersch, J. (2000) Reading the case record: The oral and written narratives of social work, *Social Services Review*, 74(2), 169–192.

Fook, J. (2002) Theorizing from practice: Towards an inclusive approach for social work research, *Qualitative Social Work*, 1(1), 79–95.

Gouldner, A. W. (1960) The norm of reciprocity: A preliminary statement, *American Sociological Review*, 25(2), 161–178.

Halvorsen, K. (1998) Symbolic purposes and factual consequences of the concepts "self-reliance and "dependency" in contemporary discourses on welfare, *Scandinavian Journal of Social Welfare*, 7, 57–65.

Houston, S. (2001) Beyond social constructionism: Critical realism and social work, *British Journal of Social Work*, 31, 845–861.

Humphries, B. (2003) What else counts as evidence in evidence-based social work? *Social Work Education*, 22(1), 81–91.

Humphries, B. (2004) Taking Sides: Research as a Moral and Political Activity. In Lovelock, R. L. (ed.), *Reflecting on Social Work-Discipline and Profession*, Aldershot: Ashgate, 113–129.

Kjørstad, M. (2008a) Administrative Discretion in Social Work: A Theoretical Approach to a Practical Matter. In Koht, H. & Tufte, G. (eds.), *Civil Society, Local Government and Human Services in the Baltic Sea Region*, Oslo: Oslo and Akershus University College, pp. 215–221.

Kjørstad, M. (2008b) Opening the black box – Mobilizing practical knowledge in social research: Methodological reflections based on a study of social work practice, *Qualitative Social Work*, 7(2), 143–161.

Kjørstad, M. (2008c) Et kritisk, realistisk perspektiv på sosialt arbeid I forvaltningen: En studie av sosialarbeideres iverksetting av arbeidslinjen i norsk sosialpolitikk [A Critical Realist Perspective on Social Work in the Public Services: A Study of Social Workers' Implementation of a Workfare Policy in Norway], Doktoravhandlinger ved NTNU 2008: 308, Norges teknisk-naturvitenskapelige universitet (NTNU).

Kjørstad, M. (2016a/2005) Between professional ethics and bureaucratic rationality: The challenging ethical position of social workers who are faced with implementing a workfare policy, *European Journal of Social Work*, 8(4), 381–398. In Shaw, I. F., Hardy, M., & Marsh, J. (2016) *Social Work Research*, Sage.

Kjørstad, M. (2016b) Do your duty – Demand your right: A theoretical discussion of the norm of reciprocity in social work, *European Journal of Social Work*, Online, November 2016

Kvale, S., & Enerstvedt, R. T. (1995) *Issues of Validity in Qualitative Research*, Lund: Studentlitteratur.

Latour, B. (1987) *Science in Action: How to Follow Scientists and Engineers Through Society*, Cambridge, MA: Harvard University Press.

Latour, B. (2000) When things strike back: A possible contribution of 'science studies' to the social sciences', *The British Journal of Sociology*, 51(1), 107–123.

Lipsky, M. (1980) *Street-Level Bureaucracy – Dilemmas of the Individual in the Public Services*, New York: Russel Sage Foundation.

Lødemel, I., & Trickey, H. (2001) *An Offer You Can't Refuse: Workfare in International Perspective*, Bristol: Policy Press.

Lundquist, L. (1988) *Byråkratisk etik [Bureaucracy ethics]*, Lund: Studentlitteratur.

Lundquist, L. (1992) *Forvaltning, stat och samhälle [The Public Services, the State and Society]*, Lund: Studentlitteratur.

Midré, G. (1995) *Bot, bedring eller brød? Om bedømming og behandling av sosial nød fra reformasjonen til velferdsstaten*, Oslo: Universitetsforlaget.

Morén, S., & Blom, B. (2003) Explaining human change: On generative mechanisms in social work practice, *Journal of Critical Realism*, 2(1), 37–60.

Pawson, R., & Tilley, N. (1997) *Realistic Evaluation*, London: Sage.

Ricoeur, P. (1981) *Hermeneutics and the Human Sciences: Essays on Language, Action and Interpretation*, Cambridge: Editions de la Maison de Sciences de l'Homme & Cambridge University Press.

Rothstein, B. (1998) *Just Institutions Matter: The Moral and Political Logic of the Universal Welfare State*, Cambridge: Cambridge University Press.

Rothstein, B. (2001) *Politik som Organisation: Förvaltningspolitikens grundproblem [Politics as Organization: The Main Problems of Public Administration Politics]*, Stockholm: SNS Förlag.

Sannerstedt, A. (2001) Implementering – hur politiska beslut genomförs i praktiken [Implementation – How Political Decisions Is Implemented in Practice]. In Rothstein, B. (ed.), *Politik som organisation: Förvaltningspolitikens grundproblem [Politics as Organization: The Main Problems of Public Administration Politics]*, Stockholm: SNS Förlag, pp. 18–48.

Sayer, A. (2000; 2008) *Realism and Social Science*, London: Sage.

Terum, L. I. (1996) *Grenser for Sosialpolitisk Modernisering [Bounderies of the Modernising of Social Politics]*, Oslo: Universitetsforlaget.

Vike, H., Bakken, R., Haukelien, H., & Kroken, R. (2002) *Maktens samvittighet: om politkk, styring og dilemmaer i velferdsstaten [The Conscience of Power: Politics, Management and Dilemmas in the Welfare State]*, Oslo: Gyldendal akademisk.

White, S. (2000) Social rights and the social contract – Political theory and the new welfare politics, *British Journal of Political Science*, 30, 533–540.

7 Encounters uncovered

Implementing critical realism and domain theory in ethnographic research with young masculinities

Harry Lunabba

Introduction

Raised by an engineer father but educated by postmodern academic scholars, I have always experienced the dilemma of fitting the subjective and objective elements of reality into a coherent understanding of social life. The implication of this dilemma for my early ethnographic fieldwork was that I was often felt anxiety about whether my observations had scientific legitimacy and whether the data enabled me to make any reliable truth claims or sufficiently thick descriptions (Geertz, 1975) of the social conduct I was observing. As a novice gender researcher, I experienced a strong sensation that I should have some kind of idea how biology or other "objective" aspects affect boys' behavior. I have also been concerned about bias and how, through my ethnographic participation, I influenced and spoiled the school settings and activities that I was supposed to impartially observe. On the other hand, being educated in social constructionist theory (Berger & Luckman, 1967; Karvinen-Niinikoski, 2009), I have gained awareness of the constructivist nature of knowledge. I am still particularly fond of the social constructivist views of childhood and how it utterly and rightfully challenges the dominant views of children (Qvortrup, 2005; Prout & James, 1997; Corsaro, 2005; Lee, 2001). Through my readings of childhood sociology, I have become convinced of how children, particularly boys, are often misinterpreted by psychologically and biologically orientated theories (Woodhead, 1997; Frosh et al., 2002).

The objective of this chapter is to discuss the implementation of critical realist theory when conducting ethnographic research. I cannot say that critical realism cured my anxieties completely or that it gave answers to all of the questions I had during my early stages as a researcher, but I believe that critical realist theory offers concepts and tools to critically examine complex social realities. Critical realist theory and domain theory, in particular, have been useful for providing ideas and concepts on how to manage and make sense of complex ethnographic data. My aim is to present how critical realist thinking can be implemented in ethnographic research, partly as a way to position ethnographic research in relation to other research methodologies (Danermark et al., 2002; Brewer, 2000). I will also discuss how implementation of critical realist thinking enables the development of analytical frames for analyzing social life in general and social encounters in particular. The discussion presented here draws on two ethnographic studies: my doctoral thesis on adults' encounters of teenage boys in school (Lunabba, 2013) and my current research project exploring welfare work and youth work with young masculinities. I regard my use of critical realist theory as creative. By refraining from positioning myself or my research in relation to strict critical realist dogma, I have allowed myself to creatively adopt ideas and concepts outside the borders of realist doctrines (such as Collins, 2004; Scheff, 1997; Goffman, 1983). I have also taken the liberty of doing this due to my understanding of critical realism as an inclusive metatheory that acknowledges both objective and subjective elements of human conduct, as well as micro and macro structures of social environments. My aim is to show through examples how critical realist theory (Bhaskar, 2008/1975; Archer, 1995; 2003) and domain theory (Layder, 2006; 1997) can be creatively applied when analyzing encounters and situated activities based on ethnographic data.

Before I get into a discussion of the implementation of theory, I will introduce the context of this discussion by presenting two studies where the critical realist–based methodology has been and is being applied and developed. The implementation of critical realist theory will be discussed in three sections. I will start by addressing my critical realist–orientated ethnographic approach when conducting fieldwork in the context of an upper-level compulsory school. The aim is to identify some key features of my methodological orientation. That will be followed by a discussion of how the use of critical realist theory (Danermark et al., 2002; Blom & Moren 2015 p. 126) and domain theory (Layder, 1993, p. 72) enabled me to position my study and narrow the analysis to a particular segment of social reality in school. Last, I will present a framework for the analysis that I intend to use in my ongoing research on encounters between young masculinities and welfare and youth work professionals.

The context of discussion

For my doctoral thesis, I conducted ethnographic fieldwork for a period of approximately nine months in two upper-level compulsory schools in Helsinki, Finland. The thesis (Lunabba, 2013) was written in Swedish, but I have published two papers in English based on the same analysis (Lunabba, 2015; 2016). The data consisted of everyday life observations of five different classes' activities (grades 7–9) during the 2008–09 school year. I encountered about 100 young people age 13–16 during the fieldwork. Interviews were conducted with 34 boys, 11 girls, and 18 adults enrolled in the school. The majority of the adults interviewed were teachers, but I also interviewed a principal, the school's social worker, a health-care professional and a school assistant. The interviews with the adults and young people were conducted in individual, pair or group settings.

My current ethnographic study consists of a research project titled *Vulnerable masculinities in the making: A study on how boys and young masculinities encounter welfare and youth work professionals.* With the concept of "young masculinities", I underline a central aspect of my orientation: understanding boys as an intersectional social category (compare Frosh et al., 2002). My aim is to address boys simultaneously from a generational and a gender perspective, recognizing them as a contemporary and distinctive social category in relation to adult masculinities or other gender groups. The study is based on ethnographic fieldwork in two settings. From September 2015 to February 2016, I participated in a weekly workshop on rap music that targets immigrant youth. The workshop, led by two musicians with a youth work-orientated approach, gathered approximately 8 to 18 young people each week to engage in writing and recording rap music. Most of the attendees visited the workshop regularly, but the group was open to everyone. During most weeks, new people came to try out the workshop. Some became regulars, but for many the workshop was only a one- or two-time experience. During my weekly visits at the workshop, I encountered about 30 attendees, approximately half of whom had an immigrant background. Ten young people were interviewed (seven boys and three girls). I also interviewed the two youth workers that led the workshop.

The second field study was conducted at a youth work centre that specialized in supporting boys and young masculinities. The House for Boys (Finnish: *Poikien Talo*) is governed by the Finnish Settlement Union and Kalliola Settlement Association. The house offers boys age 13–28 low-threshold welfare services. These services consist of various forms of individual and group activities, such as individual and group therapy, sex education and counselling, support groups for young fathers, cooking and yoga classes, various gaming groups, camps, trips and sport activities. I conducted fieldwork on Wednesday evenings, attending a so-called open group for boys. Open group evenings target boys who have experienced or have problems fitting into regular youth houses.[1] These open groups have no explicit agenda but to offer space for boys to interact with one another and get low-threshold support from adult welfare professionals. Open group activities can sometimes complement individual supportive work or other therapeutic support provided by the House for Boys or another welfare institution. Open groups can also work as accessible entry points for boys who might shy away from individual or group counselling. The boys and young masculinities that visit open evenings have various kinds of personal reasons for attending, but many of them have experienced challenges in gaining social contacts with their peers. Some have experienced bullying, while some have experiences of being isolated and lonely. Some of the boys struggle with their gender identities and some have been diagnosed with Asperger's syndrome or have autistic tendencies.

The current data consists of observations and interviews with five boys. In 2015, one year prior to my fieldwork, I conducted a group interview with the staff of the House for Boys in collaboration with a student that wrote her master's thesis on boys' vulnerability (Sällström, 2015). This group interview will also be included in the final analysis.

Uncovering the reality and the boundaries of ethnographic research

As Bhaskar (1975, p. 56) argues, and as it has been thoroughly discussed in this book, reality can be divided into three domains: the real, the actual and the empirical. Based on this view, one can assume that: 1) there is a reality that exists independently from human knowledge, 2) reality reveals itself indirectly through the actual domain, and 3) empirical observations of reality are directly dependent on the actual domain, which determines what kinds of mechanisms can be revealed or identified (Danermark et al., 2002, p. 20). The three domains – the real, actual and empirical – can be divided further. The domain of the real can be divided into social, historical, biological, chemical, physical and metaphysical domains. The actual domain can include various scientific procedures or methodological approaches, as well as situational elements such as timing, momentum or simple coincidence. The actual domain is also responsive to structural changes in society that generate shifts in power relations or societal interests. And obviously there are various ways of experiencing empirical observations, such as seeing, hearing, feeling, calculating, measuring or keeping track of time.

What this nuanced and complex, yet understandable, logic offers to ethnographers is a way of understanding how an ethnographer's empirical observations are linked to the limits of methodology, but also how ethnographic observations complement scientific or other kinds of observations and experiences of reality. In the context of a school, the social reality is everything that happens there, and that reality can be studied in various ways. Statistics and questionnaires can provide access to lots of data on several schools, allowing a researcher to compare study results (like PISA) or students' experiences of their health and welfare (Currie et al., 2008). An ethnographic study has a much more limited scope in terms of the amount of informants or the extent of schools that are analyzed. But ethnography enables researchers to analyze elements of reality that are not revealed through other research methods, like everyday life practices or sensitive issues such as boys' experiences of teachers or their supportive needs.

On a fundamental level, social life can be understood as an energy- and time-consuming human activity. But from a more practical and ethnographic point of view, everyday life in school is about human interaction, education, learning, and maintaining and building relationships. It is also about laughter and frustration, making friends, being alone, and social engagement and disengagement. An ethnographer that enters a school soon experiences the enormous amount of interaction that goes on in and outside the classroom. Ethnographers might struggle with the notion that so many of the activities will be left unnoticed, undocumented and unanalyzed (Gordon et al. 2005). To some extent, this is because of the deliberate methodological choices that ethnographers make (Brewer, 2000). However, the ethnographic scope is also limited due to such mundane aspects as personal interests, motivations and prior experiences (Agar, 1980).

Applying Bhaskar's (1975) thoughts on the transcendental nature of reality enabled me to analytically pinpoint some of the crucial elements of my methodological approach and reveal what kinds of empirical observations were actualized in my study. Brewer (2000, pp. 53–54) presents a list of these crucial elements in his thorough presentation of ground rules for realist ethnography. The list highlights how ethnographers should identify the specific topic of interest in the study, how access to the field is negotiated with keypersons, and how trust and rapport is developed with informants. Even though ethnographic research is often understood as an open-ended approach with a particular interest of describing and analyzing the broad complexities of everyday life, the ethnographer's gaze (Gordon et al., 2005) is methodologically limited and concentrated on a set number of particularities. When making claims about the social order in school, based on ethnographic observations, it is crucial that the ethnographer address what and whom has been the focus of engagement and what particular mechanisms have been actualized for empirical observations.

One central aspect that critical reflection on my research gaze made me realize was how I had mainly focused on a relatively small, hegemonic group of boys during fieldwork at the first school, whereas I had hardly engaged with or recognized silent and socially withdrawn boys. This realization enabled me to adjust my gaze when I conducted fieldwork at the second school, and it encouraged me to also include these "other boys" or "non-hegemonic" masculinities (Renold, 2004) in my analysis. In the following, I will further address what kind of observations were actualized by positioning the study on boys in school into a particular research context.

Positioning the study: focus on classroom structures and interpersonal mechanisms

Derek Layder (1993) presents a useful research map in which he points out four different levels of social research contexts, linked to what he later defines as domains of social reality (Layder, 1997; 2006). In Layder's (2006, p. 273) view, social reality is multidimensional, consisting of four interconnected domains: contextual resources, social setting, situated activity and psychobiography. The domains vary in their macro/micro scales but also in terms of the extent to which they restrict or enable individual agency. The domain of contextual resources or the domain of a wider context (see Danermark et al., 2002, pp. 168–169) consists of material and immaterial resources, aptitudes and capabilities that are unevenly allocated and distributed among individuals and social groups. Social setting outlines the immediate environments of human actions, such as formal institutes like schools or hospitals or informal environments like local settings or family and friendship networks. The domain of situated activity is closely related to Erving Goffman's (1983) interaction order, which places the focus on the immediate encounter of two or more people. Finally, the domain of psychobiography outlines the unique and subjective experiences of an individual's life course: how previous and current human relations condition individual experiences and how experiences, as well as the great narrative of a human being, are constantly redeveloped as one interacts in the social world. Even though the various domains are interconnected and cannot be separated from one another, because all aspects of social reality influence each domain, it is practically impossible to include all domains in a single study (Danermark et al., 2002, p. 169). In Figure 7.1, I try to illustrate with Layder's research map what domains of a school were investigated in my analysis of boys' social reality there.

On the left, I situate the four social domains. On the right, I place the empirical data I collected during the fieldwork. The logic is as follows. In a macro sense, schools vary in their material and immaterial resources. In the context of Finland, the variations in schools' resources may be regarded as minor, due to the Nordic welfare model (Arnesen & Lundahl, 2006). However, schools are affected by broader political aspects, such as economic cuts and variations in how education is prioritized at different times. Schools are also local social settings, with local cultures, practices and administration. The contextual resources of schools, as well as their local social setting, could be objectives for social analysis. Exploring the local setting of a school could be undertaken by an ethnographic researcher, whereas the domain of contextual resources probably calls for other kinds of methodological approaches, such as expert interviews, document analysis or statistics. In my study, however, the particular focus was on two micro domains: the social order in classrooms (which I located between the domains of social settings and situated activity) and social interplay (which I located between the domains of situated activity and psychobiography).

Locating the analysis within a particular position enabled me to narrow the analysis to a level that was manageable for analysis. Roughly two types of mechanisms and structures were scrutinized. First, the analysis revealed how various *classrooms* differ from one another in terms of their local and interpersonal structures. Boys' challenges to keep up with schoolwork, maintain good

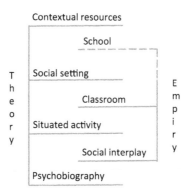

Figure 7.1 Implementation of Derek Layder's (1993) research map

behaviour or be noticed in classrooms vary in different local classroom settings (Lunabba, 2013, p. 144). The variances can be further linked to the varieties of student groups, as different student groups have different individual and interpersonal qualities. A crucial aspect of how behavioural and motivational problems are manifested is to what extent the classroom environment reaches a state of relational convergence. The term "convergence" refers to a state of emotional attunement (Scheff, 1997) or trust, as well as how much teachers and students in a particular class reach a level of collaboration and joint action. This leads to the conclusion that many of the boys' challenges in school are not objective in terms of particular disorders and disabilities, but contextually dependent on the social classroom setting, particularly the state of the social bond between adults in school and boys. Identification of boys' problems and need of support are also often relationship-based rather than determined by standardized means or objective assessments (Lunabba, 2015).

Second, the analysis aims to uncover what kinds of *interpersonal* mechanisms define the various relationships between adults and boys, as well as to uncover boys' psychobiographic experiences of their encounters with adults. In the analysis, I identified three elements in social interplay that define a relationship.[2] *Insight* refers to the informational aspect in a relationship: what one knows about the other in terms of prior life events, but also in terms of the ability to gain access to one another's subjective experiences and personal traits. I argue that a relationship between a teacher and a student can be valued by the extent to which a teacher has access to: 1) information and insight about a student's previous life patterns, 2) information and insight about a student's possible and desirable future trajectories and 3) information and insight about how a student responds in changing and emerging contextual situations (Lunabba, 2016, p. 102).

The concept *influence* refers to how power dynamics constrain or enable meaningful interaction between two parties: namely, to what extent a teacher can be effective in his or her communication with students. In Layder's (2009, p. 52) terms, a crucial element in human interaction is what he calls benign control – the power element that enables people to influence each other. Influence can be further linked to both categorical and subjective aspects (Goffman, 1983). A teacher or a social worker can make an impact based on their categorical position in a school setting and based on categorical teaching skills and knowledge. However, influence also includes subjective mechanisms like charisma, charm or whatever factors make a teacher likeable, trustworthy and inspirational. Finally, *emotion* can be regarded as the key element to define varieties in different relationships. I found Randall Collins' (2004) concept of emotional energy to be a useful concept, because emotional energy can vary in its intensity (high and low) and it can also vary in terms of its characteristics (positive or negative).

By elaborating on the three concepts that frame a relationship between an adult and a teenage boy, I was able to identify three groups of boys whose problems and needs of support often fell outside the gaze of teachers and other adults working at the school. The category *boys who are not taken seriously* refers to the widely reported discourse of how boys' underachievement, bad behaviour or lack of interest in literacy is something typical and unavoidable, given boys' "universal nature" (Lunabba, 2015; Epstein et al., 1998; Gilbert & Gilbert, 1998; Pollack, 1999; Foster et al., 2001; Young & Bronzo, 2001). The category *boys who evoke negative emotions* refers to the tendency of how boys' visible and extroverted behaviour is often interpreted through a pre-assumptive negative framework (Lunabba, 2015, p. 73). Negatively charged pre-assumptions about loud and dominant boys in class do not always encourage adults to recognize the boys' individual challenges, because the focus is more often on how loud boys are a problem for others or how adults lack influence over troubled boys. The category *boys who do not evoke emotions* highlights the mechanism by which some boys maintain invisibility in school and are not targeted with support or teachers' concerns. A common way of understanding invisibility in school is that it is especially the silent and withdrawn students that are invisible (Gordon et al., 2005). However, what I found in interviews was that both students and teachers reflected on the well-being of the silent students in particular and were especially concerned about overly silent boys. These boys seemed to generate strong emotions among their peers and teachers, which manifested as concern, pity and anxiety. The silent boys were not unrecognized, because they evoked emotions in their surroundings. Further analysis showed that invisibility among boys is more about the state of the pupils in between the overly silent students and dominant, loud students. These are boys who appear average and do not dominate the classroom in a positive or negative way. Students and teachers, as well as ethnographic researchers in classrooms, seldom direct their gaze at them, assuming that they are doing just fine. Nevertheless, in reality, most really do not know how they are doing (Lunabba, 2015, p. 76).

Re-framing situated reality and meaningfulness encounters

The focus of my ongoing research project is to explore young masculinities in the context of welfare and youth work. The research project targets two questions. The first objective is to analyze the varieties of masculine vulnerability: *how is masculine vulnerability conditioned[3] and experienced within the context of youth and welfare work?* The second objective is to further explore the situated activity (Layder, 2006, 277) when young masculinities encounter adults: *how are rapport, trust and attunement generated in the interplay between young masculinities and professional youth and welfare workers?* In my previous work, I was mainly engaged with the mechanism of how boys are recognized in school and how relationships affect how boys' problems are interpreted and constructed. My current interest is on the micro-context of the actual encounter between a boy and a youth work or welfare work professional. I am particularly interested in analyzing what generates meaningfulness in a setting where a boy's needs and problems are encountered. I use the concept of meaningfulness as a supplement for what in evidence-based practice is often referred to as "effect" (Webb, 2001; McNeece & Thyer, 2004). The connotative difference is that, whereas effect refers to the efficiency of a method or approach, I understand meaningfulness as referring to the efficiency of the method and approach in combination with individual, emotional and social elements. My pre-assumption is that a method can be proven to be effective, but in a particular contextual setting, it may lack effect or be experienced as useless, not due to the method itself, but due to other elements, such as individual, emotional or social factors.

In my previous study, I implemented domain theory mainly to generate a model for distinguishing macro school settings from local and situational classroom settings and various interpersonal settings. For the analysis of encounters and relationships, I mainly implemented interactionist theories such as Goffman's (1983) interaction order and Scheff's (1997) theory of social bonds. This new model is mostly inspired by Layder's (2009) work on intimate relationships. Layder acknowledges five energizing games in personal relationships that correspond to basic human needs: 1) the mutual seduction game refers to humans' basic need to be loved, accepted and approved; 2) the identity-affirming game corresponds to every person's need to be recognized as a unique individual; 3) the empathy game parallels the human need to be emotionally understood; 4) the altruistic game refers to the efforts needed to maintain engagement in relationships; and 5) the mutually supportive game refers to the dynamic balance of supporting dependency on one another and maintaining individual independence from one another.

A further aim of the model is that it should correspond to the complexity of the social university and acknowledge how professional encounters include objective, subjective, individual and collective dimensions and mechanisms. In Figure 7.2, I illustrate the four dimensions of energizing games included in

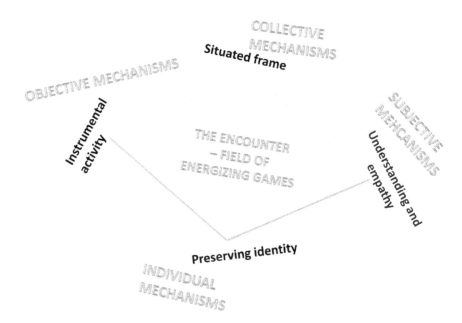

Figure 7.2 Energizing games in professional encounters

the analysis. The social universe is understood as multidimensional, consisting of both objective and subjective elements (Bhaskar (2008/1975, pp. 22–24), as well as individual and collective dimensions (Archer, 1995, pp. 42–54). Another aim is to grasp the depth of a particular encounter without losing sight of the objective, subjective, individual and collective elements. In other words, my aim is to adhere to realist theory and domain theory, even though I also include ideas from other theoretical traditions, such as interaction theories and theories of social bonds.

Objective and subjective mechanisms in social interplay

In Bhaskar's (2008/1975, p. 22) terms, there are two sides of knowledge: one that refers to the subjective and socially constructed experiences of individuals and one that refers to the knowledge of objects that exist regardless of human awareness. The encounter being in all of its aspects human activity, all of its elements fall into the wide range of transformed and constructed knowledge, which exists because of human conduct. What I refer to in Figure 7.2 as the *objective mechanism* cannot therefore be regarded as objective in the sense what Bhaskar refers to as the real, ontological or intransitive dimension of reality (Bhaskar, 2008/1975, p. 24). The notion of objective mechanisms is more about the epistemological paradigm that idealizes antecedent science models: the established facts and theories, models and techniques that welfare workers and youth workers may apply in their professional conduct. The most practical way of understanding the objective mechanisms in Figure 7.2 is how it represents a counterpart to the *subjective mechanisms*. Whereas objective mechanisms can be regarded as the somewhat fixed routines or science-based methods and knowledge-based models that are implemented in professionals' encounters with young people, subjective mechanisms refer to the range of individual and emotional experiences involved in human interplay. In my understanding of the subjective mechanism, I lean on Margaret Archer's (2003, p. 153) thinking and what she refers to as internal conversations – the sources of variations in people's thinking. When examining human interplay from these two dimensions, the objective mechanisms highlight the sufficiency of established routines in a variety of human encounters. The subjective mechanisms correspond to the particular interests and emotional needs of a particular individual in a given situation.

The concept of *instrumental activity* is linked to the epistemology of objective mechanisms that occur in a welfare or youth work setting where professionals encounter young people. Each professional encounter has some kind of main purpose linked to a professional objective and to professionally motivated or expected practices and procedures. These professional activities can be regarded as the instrumental, main reasons for any professional conduct and the response to formal expectations of any kind of professional welfare or youth work. For instance, when I interviewed young people who participated in the rap workshop, the obvious and crucial aspects of the workshop for most of the young people were the workshop leaders' skills and talent as rap musicians. When asked about what they valued in the workshop, it was evident that the first aspects that young people reflected on were the professional abilities and the core activity of music.

Ip2A: Aleksi likes making the beats. He does, well, that's his strength. He makes the beat for us. And Shaka helps us with our writing.

Harry: So how do they help you? What do they do? What helps?

Ip2A: Well. If someone, like, needs help with their lyrics, Shaka can, like, open things up. He knows what's good, you know. And he can, like, say what you need to change or fix to make it work. Shaka is good, you know, and he can teach. He knows his stuff.

The dimension of instrumental activity can be understood as the objective, knowledge-based aspect in a professional encounter. It can refer to both the technical skills of a musician handling an instrument and the professional, science-based skills of a welfare worker. It is evident in music-making that musicians have different levels of skill, which can be evaluated in somewhat objective terms. For instance, *Aleksi* – who produced, edited and recorded the rap music created at the workshop – was admirably skillful at producing and creating beats. Frankly, I was astonished how rapidly he could create, every week, an original rap beat in a timespan of half an hour, using Logic Pro software or some other music sampler. *Shaka*, being a recording artist, also had obvious skills and talent in writing and performing rap music, and he had the legitimacy to give constructive criticism to workshop participants. Welfare workers' skills are perhaps not that evident, but I would claim that some instrumental techniques and working models for human interaction are more efficient than others. The aspects of how welfare professionals initiate conversations, how they can apply suitable approaches and models with various people, or how they can generate the sensation of an energy-charging atmosphere are to an extent dependent on the professional's skills. One objective of my ethnographic exploration of youth workers and welfare workers' encounters with young masculinities is to understand what kinds of approaches and work skills are experienced as effective. However, acknowledging that young masculinities are a complex and multidimensional social category, it is not my intention to suggest that a specific method or model is most effective with masculinities. The idea is rather to identify young masculinities and youth workers' views on what counts as skillful in a general sense (compare Lefevre, 2010, pp. 25–42).

As stated earlier, there is more to an encounter than skills and methods. On the opposite side of instrumental activity is the dimension of subjective mechanisms. In my analysis, I have operationalized this side of social reality as the concepts *understanding* and *empathy*. This dimension refers to the varieties of emotional and informative connections in human encounters. As Archer (2003, p. 167) describes, everyone has a domain of mental privacy from which they subjectively operate in relation to their surroundings. For this dimension, however, I prefer to rely on Thomas J. Scheff's (1997, p. 76) concept of attunement, which refers to mutual identification and understanding in the interplay of two or more individuals. People find themselves in youth work settings and welfare work institutions for various reasons and they can appreciate various kinds of skills and the personal traits of a professional. However, what was often mentioned by young people I encountered during my research project is the importance of being understood. This aspect has both the dimension of being understood on an informative level and the dimension of being emotionally connected (Lunabba, 2016). Not reaching out to one another or not being fully or sufficiently understood is an energy-draining sensation, which by all means can be linked to a professional's communication skills. However, the dimension of understanding and empathy refers to the encountering parties' subjectivity and reflective capacities (Archer, 2003, pp. 170–176; 214–220) and how human beings as subjects engage in different ways with different kinds of people. In simple terms, people have various kinds of interests and desires. As I found when exploring the relationships of adults and boys in school, the subjectivity of a human being can sometimes be manifested as an objective inability to attune, due to differences with individuals' interpersonal chemistry (Lunabba, 2013, p. 175). Exploring the emotionality in how and with whom young masculinities connect may reveal some of the challenges of welfare and youth work that are linked to the uniqueness of individuals and to the eventual particularities of young masculinities.

Individual and collective mechanisms in social interplay

In my understanding of individual and collective mechanisms in human interplay, I mainly rely on Archer's (1995, p. 33) argument that "neither Individualism nor Collectivism can furnish the basis for adequate social theorizing". Individual mechanisms and collective mechanisms that are included in the previous model are understood as interwoven dimensions influencing one another, and therefore they cannot be separated in social analysis. Individuals' identities are generated, challenged and re-affirmed in social situations with others. Social groups, cultures and social situations are a result of individuals' social engagements. When interpreting the meanings of human conduct within the frame of a particular situated activity, one can build arguments about how individuals tend to present themselves to one another based on individuals' unique psychobiographic identities (Layder, 2006, p. 274) or iterations (Emirbayer & Mische, 1998, p. 970). On the contrary, social analysis has revealed how the momentum or the particularity of a situation can generate extraordinary human behaviour that can be contradictory to an individual's previous behavioural patterns, habits or self-identity. As Goffman (2005/1967, p. 3) explains, "Not then, men and their moments. Rather, moment and their men." This viewpoint also corresponds to the structure agency dilemma, which is one of the key debates in critical realism (Layder, 2006; Archer, 1995; Bhaskar, 1986). Identities as well as situations are understood because of two phenomena. On the one hand, both identities and situations are a result of enabling or constraining *social structures*. However, situations and identities are also maintained, reproduced and transformed through the activities of *social agents* (Danermark et al. 2002, p. 180). This thought process resolves in a viewpoint that highlights how social realties are dynamic. Identities and situations where welfare professionals encounter young professionals are constantly shifting. Identities are being preserved and situations are being framed.

The third aspect under scrutiny in the study, *preserving identity*, is how encounters in youth and welfare work can challenge young masculinities' identities. The operationalization of the individual mechanisms aims to highlight on one hand the uniqueness of a particular boy, but at the same time it acknowledges how boys' identities are enabled and constrained by social structures and norms. A lot has been said about boys and young masculinities' inabilities or challenges to engage with supporters and caregivers, and one way to articulate this is how welfare settings may drain or threaten masculine identities. It has been claimed that boys and young masculinities lack the ability or permission to express vulnerability and that this could explain the challenge to reach out to boys (Salisbury & Jackson, 1996, p. 24; Pascoe, 2007, pp. 50–59). The dimension of preserving identity aims to target the mechanisms of identity work involved in human interplay. The notion is to acknowledge how human psychobiography is unique due to individuals' various life courses and relationships (Layder, 2006, p. 274). But in reference to Bhaskar's (1986, pp. 129–136) transformative model of human action, individuals' psychobiographies are also transformed or re-charged by new social encounters and relationships. The identities or the unique psychobiography of an individual can in a sense be updated as a result of successful energy-charging identity work during a social encounter. Encounters and social interplay can also challenge or threaten identities to the extent that all available energy is directed toward preserving and protecting the self (Layder, 1997, pp. 67–72). In exploring the dimension of preserving identity, the aim is to reveal the mechanisms of how identities are preserved and developed in the course of youth and welfare work. A further aim is to also explore if or how contemporary masculine identities hinder boys and young men from engaging in supportive youth and welfare work. According to *interview person 1*, a young man age 24, the discourse that prevents a boy from expressing emotions still exists, but it did not apply to him personally.

Ip1: This might just be my experience, but there is that idea that you should be, like, kind of formed a certain way. That you should be like a tough dude. And then you should not, like, show your feelings. There is that kind of a problem [being a young masculinity].

Harry: I wanted to ask, do you somehow have to relate to this stereotype? Do you have to hide your feelings or be in a certain way?

Ip1: No. I have decided that I'm not gonna be that guy.

Finally, the analysis focuses on exploring the *situated framing* of the context where particular encounters take place. With the situated frame, I refer to Goffman's (1983) interaction order. In domain theory, the momentum that occurs between the beginning and the end of an encounter is referred to as situated activity (Layder, 2006, p. 177). What both Layder's and Goffman's work indicate is that this situated micro setting can be stretched out both in time and space and linked to various layers of the social universe. In this particular analysis, however, my aim is to focus on the specific inputs and outputs of participants in an encounter. The viewpoint highlights how every encounter occurs in a situated frame that is directly linked to immediate engagements and reactions of the interplay between two or more parts (even though it also extends to wider social structures, such as the institutional structures of social work and youth work organizations, as well as the structures that enable or hinder boys' engagement in supportive social work). During research with young masculinities, I have experienced how the micro settings have a tendency to be overly positive (nothing is taken seriously) or overly negative (responses to engagement are unkind, insulting or dismissive). As *Shaka* reflects, as a workshop leader he needs to make an effort to maintain a positive and constructive atmosphere that allows and encourages participants to create and perform in the group.

Shaka: What seems to be, like, common among boys is that habit that you always, like, mock one another.

Harry: Sounds kind of familiar.

Shaka: I still have friends who, like, interact in their everyday life like this. They don't necessarily intend to be mean to one another. It's more like a habit. But that is, like, something we've tried to avoid here in our interplay. Even though that kind of interaction occurs elsewhere, this setting would be, like, free from it. 'Cause if you, like, don't really intend to be, like, mean it still keeps people on their toes. Like if I know that if I say something embarrassing that that other guy will mock me, in the worst case, like maybe next week. Like, put me again in that embarrassing spot. So everything can be the kind of stuff that someone can use to tease me and expose my emotions or thoughts or something about myself. And why we, like, try to weed out that kind of behaviour from these sessions is that that would not, like, ever occur here. We have not, like, been totally successful in weeding it out. But in general terms, I think we have succeeded in making this atmosphere that is safe and supportive. And it's not, like, common that people mock each other here.

In a previous article, I also reflected on how I needed to make an effort to create a serious enough atmosphere during interviews with teenage boys (Lunabba, 2016). The dimension of the situated framework complements the analysis by scrutinizing the subtle but significant varieties in engagements and responses in specific encounters, and furthermore it explores how secure social bonds are created with young masculinities: bonds that are neither too tight (negative) nor too loose (nothing is taken seriously) (Scheff, 1997, p. 77). In brief, the aim is to acknowledge the situational context when determining the effectiveness and meaningfulness of an encounter. In Bhaskar's (1986, p. 131) terms, it is about acknowledging how immediate social structures condition social activity but structures are at the same time a direct result of participants' engagement with and responses to one another.

Conclusion

In this chapter, I have discussed how I have implemented critical realist thinking in my ethnographic work. The views and ideas that have been presented are not based on a dogmatic use of critical realist theory, but a creative one. This chapter is not intended to be a textbook example of how critical realist theory or domain theory should be used in ethnographic research. It is more of an example of how it can be used in creative combination with other social theories that address various mechanisms in human encounters. Critical realism offers concepts of how an ethnographic researcher may relate to other research methods or methodologies, as well as ideas of how to position ethnographic conduct in a complex yet manageable social universe. The use of critical realist theory, as well as the use of well-thought-out abstractions of the social universe, distinguishes systematic ethnography from laypersons' observations (Brewer, 2000, p. 55). Above all, critical realist theory offers the researcher ways to organize and systematically examine complex and nuanced research data.

Notes

1 Youth houses in Finland are often organized by municipalities. They offer after-school activities and spaces for leisure time for children and young people.
2 The three elements are based on Mustafa Emirbayer and Ann Mische's (1998, p. 970) theoretical work on the chordal triad of agency.
3 By "condition", I refer to the work of Margaret Archer (Archer, 1995, pp. 54–61).

References

Agar, M. H. (1980) *The Professional Stranger: An Informal Introduction to Ethnography*, New York: Academic Press.

Archer, M. S. (1995) *Realist Social Theory: The Morphogenetic Approach*, Cambridge: Cambridge University Press.

Archer, M. S. (2003) *Structure, Agency and Internal Conversation*, Cambridge: Cambridge University Press.

Arnesen, A-L., & Lundahl, L. (2006) Still social and democratic? Inclusive education policies in the Nordic welfare states, *Scandinavian Journal of Educational Research*, 50(3), 285–300.

Berger, P., & Luckman, T. (1967) *The Social Construction of Reality: A Treatise of in the Sociology of Knowledge*, New York: Doubleday.

Bhaskar, R. (1986) *Scientific Realism and Human Emancipation*, London: Verso.

Bhaskar, R. (2008/1975) *A Realist Theory of Science*, London: Verso Books.

Blom, B., & Morén, S. (2015) *Teori för socialt arbete*, Lund: Studentlitteratur.

Brewer, J. D. (2000) *Ethnography*, Buckingham: Open University Press.

Collins, R. (2004) *Interaction Ritual Chains*, Princeton, NJ: Princeton University Press.

Corsaro, W. A. (2005) *The Sociology of Childhood*, Thousand Oaks, CA: Pine Forge.

Currie, C., Gabhainn, S. N., Godeau, E., Roberts, C., Smith, R., Currie, D., Picket, W., Richter, M., Morgan, A., & Barnekow, V. (2008) *Inequalities in Young People's Health: HBSC International Report From the 2005/2006 Survey*, Edinburgh: World Health Organization.

Danermark, B., Ekström, M., Jakobsen, L., & Karlsson, J. Ch. (2002) *Explaining Society*, London: Routledge.

Emirbayer, M., & Mische, A. (1998) What is agency? *American Journal of Sociology*, 103(4). 962–1023.

Epstein, D., Elwood, J., Hey, V., & Maw, J. (1998) Schoolboy Frictions: Feminism and "Failing" Boys. In Epstein, D., Elwood, J., Hey, V., & Maw, J. (eds.), *Failing Boys? Issues in Gender and Achievement*, Buckingham: Open University Press, pp. 3–18.

Foster, V., Kimmel, M., & Skelton, C. (2001) 'What About the Boys?' An Overview of the Debates. In Martina, W. & Meyenn, B. (eds.), *What About the Boys?* Buckingham: Open University Press, pp. 1–23.

Frosh, S., Phoenix, A., & Pattman, R. (2002) *Young Masculinities: Understanding Boys in Contemporary Society*, Houndmills: Palgrave Macmillan.

Geertz, C. (1975) Thick Description: Toward an Interpretive Theory of Culture. In Geerz, C. (ed.), *The Interpretation of Cultures*, London: Hutchinson, pp. 3–32.

Gilbert, R., & Gilbert, P. (1998) *Masculinity Goes to School*, London: Routledge.

Goffman, E. (1983) *The Interaction Order*. American Sociological Association, 1982 Presidential Address, New York: American Sociological Association.

Goffman, E. (2005/1967) *Interaction Ritual: Essays in Face-to-Face Behavior*, New Brunswick, NJ: Transaction Publishers.

Gordon, T., Holland, J., Lahelma, E., & Tolonen, T. (2005) Gazing with intent: Ethnographic practice in classrooms, *Qualitative Research*, 5(1), 113–131.

Karvinen-Niinikoski, S. (2009) Postmoderni sosiaalityö. In Mäntysaari, M., Pohjola, A., & Pösö, T. (eds.), *Sosiaalityö ja teoria*, Jyväskylä: Juva, pp. 131–160.

Layder, D. (1993) *New Strategies in Social Research: An Introduction and Guide*, Cambridge: Polity Press.

Layder, D. (1997) *Modern Social Theory: Key Debates and New Directions*, London: Routledge.

Layder, D. (2006) *Understanding Social Theory* (2nd edn), London: Sage.

Layder D. (2009) *Intimacy and Power: The Dynamics of Personal Relationships in Modern Society*, Hampshire: Palgrave Macmillan.

Lee, N. (2001) *Childhood and Society: Growing up in an Age of Uncertainty*, Buckingham: Open University Press.

Lefevre, M. (2010) *Communicating With Children and Young People – Making a Difference*, Bristol: Policy Press.

Lunabba, H. (2013) *När vuxna möter pojkar i skolan – Insyn, inflytande och sociala relationer*, Helsingfors: FSKC/ Mathilda Wrede Institutet.

Lunabba, H. (2015) Recognizing Boys From an Emotional and Relational Perspective. In Hällgren, C., Dunkels, E., & Frånberg G-M. (eds.), *Invisible Boy: The Making of Contemporary Masculinities*, Umeå: Umeå University, pp. 69–78.

Lunabba, H. (2016) Exploring Relationships Through Ethnography. In Ruch, G. & Juklkunen, I. (eds.), *Relationship-Based Research in Social Work*, London: Jessica Kingsley Publishers, pp. 89–106.

McNeese, A., & Thyer, B. (2004) Evidence-based practice in social work, *Journal of Evidence-Based Social Work*, 1(1), 7–25.

Pascoe, C. J. (2007) *Dude You're a Fag: Masculinity and Sexuality in High School*, Berkley, CA: University of California Press.

Pollack, W. (1999) *Real Boys*, New York: Henry Holt and Company.

Prout, A., & James, A. (1997) A New Paradigm for the Sociology of Childhood. In James, A. & Prout, A. (eds.), *Constructing and Reconstructing Childhood: Contemporary Issues in the Sociological Study of Childhood*, London: Routledge Falmer, pp. 7–32.

Qvortrup, J. (2005) Varieties of Childhood. In Qvortrup, J. (ed.), *Studies in Modern Childhood: Society, Agency, Cultures*, Basingstoke: Palgrave Macmillan, pp. 1–20.

Renold, E. (2004) 'Other' boys: Negotiating non-hegemonic masculinities in the primary school, *Gender & Education*, 16(2), 247–266.

Salisbury, J., & Jackson, D. (1996) *Challenging Macho Values: Practical Ways of Working With Adolescent Boys*, London: Falmer Press.

Sällström, R (2015) *"Den här klumpen har funnits redan länge i hjärtat och den blir bara större" – En fallstudie om hur manlig sårbarhet kommer till uttryck i förhållande till förväntningar om maskulinitet*, Helsingfors: Helsingfors universitet.

Scheff, T. (1997) *Emotions, the Social Bond, and Human Reality: Part/Whole Analysis*, Cambridge: Cambridge University Press.

Webb, S. (2001) Some considerations on the validity of evidence-based practice in social work, *British Journal of Social Work*, 31, 57–79.

Woodhead, M. (1997) Psychology and the Cultural Constructions of Children's Needs. In James, A. & Prout, A. (eds.), *Constructing and Reconstructing Childhood: Contemporary Issues in the Sociological Study of Childhood*, London: Routledge Falmer, pp. 63–84.

Young, J. P., & Brozo, W. G. (2001) Boys will be boys, or will they? *Literacy and Masculinities: Reading Research Quarterly*, 36(3), 316–325.

8 Parenting stress and coping practices in a critical realist perspective

May-Britt Solem

This chapter addresses the relevance of using critical realism (CR) as a theory of science together with a mixed methods design in a research study of parenting stress and coping practices (Solem, 2011). The aim of the study was to broaden our understanding of parents' coping practices in families with children who have behavioural problems. I explored parents' everyday lives and their ways of under-standing, acting and interacting with a specific boy in the family. This approach addressed a gap in prior knowledge by analysing parents' coping practices in a comprehensive and nuanced way most useful in clinical practice, where social constraints together with a focus on parent-child interactions and normal family processes is taken into account. I was interested in conducting a deeper analysis of the narratives of each of the individuals (parents) involved, but I also wanted to explain and understand mechanisms in the contexts of families' everyday prac-tices. These causal mechanisms cannot be revealed directly but can be inferred through a combination of data investigation and theory building or construction.

CR emphasises that there is a mutual relationship between parental agency and structure; thus, the social contexts are constituted and influenced by parents' meaningful actions and interactions. In this understanding, both purpose-oriented actions and habitual actions are parts of parents' repertoires in everyday actions and interactions. CR supports context-sensitive analyses that explore parents' various ways of dealing with their children and their general and specific reasons for doing so. By shifting the focus from children with behavioural problems and symptoms and demanding children toward demanding situations, the meanings of age, gender, class, social support and parental resources became important in the understanding of framing family life. I see parents' practices as embedded in material, social and cultural contexts, as situated parenting, expressed through the organising of daily life. Different parents carry different cultural, biological and social possibilities and constraints, and I wanted to study the extent to which the domains restrict or enable parents' agency. I emphasised family practices from an everyday life perspective, informed by a systemic understanding of the biologi-cal, psychological and social domains involved. CR, with its focus on reality as open systems, with a multi-causal view of reality as differentiated and stratified, enabled me to take this complexity (actor and context) seriously into the analysis with an interdisciplinary approach.

I analysed the parents' narratives regarding their everyday life, and the mechanisms in play in the relationship between parenting stress, resources, coping and different risk factors. Explaining from a critical realist perspective involves describing and comprehending the mechanisms that generate and enable events in parenting practices, together with a focus on parents' coping and meaning making; this is because, according to a critical relist understanding, all people are intentional actors (Danermark et al., 2003; Sayer, 2010). CR's mechanism explanations within the social work field weigh heavily on meaning and meaning making. People make meaning of their experiences and the larger social context impinges on those meanings. According to Collins et al. (2010), we need to know more about "why" certain coping strategies are used, "when" they are used, and "when/why" they do or do not work. I also add the question of "how" to this list. Explorations of "how" parents perceive their interaction with their children in everyday life situations will be my point of departure when seeking answers to "why", which alludes to the parents' processes of making meaning in family interactions. Parents' interactions are not understood sufficiently if their intentions are not taken into account in studying parenting.

When I started with my studies there were few existing studies that had focused on parents' meaning making in "normal" or common parenting processes, as opposed to meaning making constructed of parents having children with behaviour problems. The available theory and evidence from the stress and coping literature says little about the contextual and situational influences or about parents' reflexive thinking or meaning making about their experiences with their child (Collins et al., 2010). Stress research in the social sciences has long held the promise of understanding individual and family coping and adaptation, but this knowledge has not yet informed clinical practice. Attachment concepts in psychology, however, have influenced family therapy in recent years. Family studies have become increasingly multidisciplinary, yet the bridge between the social sciences and the clinical field still needs to be widened to facilitate better exchange of perspectives on and approaches to understanding family functioning (Walsh, 2003). This brought me to the "interaction" concept, which regards children as having interaction problems and parents as having interaction repertoires with which to help their children in everyday life.

In the first section of this article, I present the results from the quantitative studies. The results revealed mechanisms that influence parenting stress in the parenting situations. Some results were unexpected and incoherent, so I went further by exploring this phenomenon qualitatively in the second section. In the third section, I address critical realism as a guided principle for the research process, and in the fourth section, I argue for a broad understanding and link to contexts in social research. In the end, I focus on the importance of mixed methods design and interdisciplinary research when studying family processes with growing diversity and complexity of families, which makes it imperative to examine the social constructs of "normality".

Parenting stress analysed in the quantitative studies

The quantitative focus of the analysis was, first, to examine parenting practices as situation-specific and analyse whether there were differences between parental conditions in parent-child interaction situations in the clinical and comparison groups. Second, I wanted to explore predictors to parenting stress as family demographics, child's behaviour problems, parents' resources and capacities.

The data contained 64 parents of boys (6–12 years) with behavioural problems (clinical group) and 128 parents of boys with fewer or no problems (comparison group). Altogether, 192 parents completed questionnaires and all of these parents were interviewed about their everyday lives. In recent years, only sparse research information has been available connecting difficult tasks in parenting to situation-specific coping capacities. In the two quantitative studies, the questionnaires focused on specific child-rearing situations and in relation to a specific child in the family.

The results showed that having a child with behaviour problems explained 57 percent of the variance in parenting stress, and social support and parental resources and strategies added to the explanation of parenting stress after controlling for family demographics and child characteristics. The most unexpected results were the prevalence of different risk factors in the clinical group compared to the comparison group. The parents in the clinical group were more often single parents with lower education, were more often unemployed, perceived less content with social support, and had lower scores on comprehensibility of their sons' behaviour. They were significantly more stressed than parents in the comparison group. They struggled not only with the children's problems but also with bad living conditions. All these different risk factors, combined with the children's symptoms, were mechanisms that influenced the parents' stress in parenting situations. The mechanisms in the parenting situation in clinical group contributed to stress and increased isolation, and the parents often became exhausted.

On the other side, there were no significant differences between the groups in terms of parents' coping capacities. How was it possible that the parents in the clinical group had significantly more risk factors in their lives than the comparison group, and at the same time did not show significant differences in coping practices? The retroductive framework enabled me to reveal the multidimensional factors involved in this inconsistency. Identifying the causal mechanisms in the realm of the real revealed the extent to which socio-economic, cultural and biological components feature in the way in which parents' interactions are assessed. I found it interesting to examine the explicit and implicit assumptions about "family normality" and extend our understanding of parent-child interactions in everyday family life. It became important and interesting to identify the diversity of the processes of family routines, values and challenges in everyday life, and to explore the processes that are typical for different families in different contexts. Research in the field of parenting often defines parental coping strategies as dysfunctional when the parents have children with disabilities. In particular, avoidance coping is understood as dysfunctional (Lloyd & Hastings, 2008). I wanted to explore parents' coping practices in both the clinical and the comparison group and to challenge whether different discourses prevailed in the two groups.

CR inspired me to try to identify social inequalities in health, both oppressive mechanisms and mechanisms that lead to well-being for different groups.

Parents' meaning making analysed in the qualitative studies

Because of the unexpected lack of significant differences between the groups regarding parents' coping practices, the next step was to explore qualitatively parents' meaning making in parent-child interactions and to challenge the main-stream treatment of avoidance actions as dysfunctional in research studies in contrast to active coping. Sixteen families were selected according to variations in marital status, age and level of the problems of the child. Families from both groups were selected.

Through the inductive analytic process, organising of family life and especially parent-child interactions emerged as important themes to pursue. In order to assess whether the lack of differences between the groups could be explained by the situational focus on the parents, avoidance actions became the initial guiding principle of the deductive analysis. Parents obviously withdrew in some way or another from time to time; after reading through and systematising the material several times, I became aware of the parents' efforts to organise family life in ways that served to avoid demanding interactions between parents and children. The CR perspective led me to analyse and develop new understandings and relations that did not emerge from the empirical data alone but also through available theory and evidence from the stress and coping literature. I found that avoidance strategies also emerged in normal family processes.

This awareness by help of an abductive process, where I alternated between relevant theory and empirical data in the analysis, led to the development of an analytic model that highlighted the mechanisms explaining parents' efforts to organise family life to avoid demanding interactions between parents and children. This model, constructed from the empirical data and the sociocultural understanding of social practices, contained three themes: (1) avoiding conflicts ("it is about framing"), (2) choosing when to intervene and (3) withdrawing to reflect on the next step. All these themes highlight the many ways in which parents avoid the construction and/or escalation of stressful interactional situations in all families (Solem, 2013a).

All parents used different ways of avoiding, ignoring or withdrawing, and these ways have to be understood in the contexts in which they were used, and why they were applied, to assess whether they were relevant or appropriate in special situations. When these avoidance actions were analysed holistically with the repertoire the parents had, they could also be seen as proactive actions and interactions. Parental practices cannot be studied in isolation, but only as situated practice where they are embedded, meaning interplays between structure and actors (Archer, 1995), more as a strong view toward inseparability (Rogoff, 1990; 1997).

The qualitative studies challenged the unbalanced focus on children's problems or symptoms and diagnoses in child and adolescent psychiatry, without taking into account the children's total life situations. A more holistic investigation around the families' living conditions is necessary to understand the children's problems or symptoms. Interdisciplinary research corresponds well to clinical practice, in which the everyday reality facing clinicians is that they must confront the "whole" complex phenomenon.

It became important to narrate how families' lives and everyday life practices were experienced for those who were striving to capture the mechanisms involved. The mixed methods design made it possible to further investigate unexpected results from the quantitative analysis; that the parents significantly experienced less social support than the comparison group while, at the same time, no significant differences between the groups regarding coping strategies were confirmed. In the qualitative analysis, issues of shame and guilt in parenting in the clinical group emerged from the abductive and retroductive analyses. The deeper focus as an abduction process, and also in a way a retroduction process, made it possible to identify mechanisms as parents' feelings of shame and guilt. Some parents reported in the interviews that they were ashamed of their child's behaviour in front of other people, which led them to avoid some potentially embarrassing social and family settings. A lot of work was involved from some of the single mothers in trying to be "an ordinary" family. The question was which possibilities the parents had, given their difficult situations. It became clear that some parents needed guided participation in the parenting situation in addition to practical and social support.

The quantitative and qualitative approaches served different purposes in this work and helped to illuminate different aspects of the studied phenomena. The quantitative approach helped to describe the relationship between stress and parenting, whereas the qualitative approach provided information about possible reasons for these interactions and actions, in terms of the actors' interpretations of situations and their goals and preferences. Both methods helped to answer different questions: the results of statistical analyses indicated the kinds of actions parents typically performed, while the analysis of the qualitative data helped answer "why" and "how" questions.

Critical realism as a guided principle for research processes

My position as a family therapist made me curious about parenting practices with challenges in interactions with their children. CR offered me a stratified ontology that made me see reality as hierarchically ordered levels that also may serve as a map for the systematic investigations of family therapy planning. By using specific theories and methods developed for each level, the results may be integrated in an attempt to reach a more holistic perspective of the phenomenon. Specific disciplines usually focus on generative mechanisms at specific levels. In my CR research process, different levels in the analysis were treated, and went beyond disciplinary limits to offer an approach that yields knowledge suited for transformation into practice. This stands in marked contrast to research that focuses on mechanisms at single levels. Also, according to critical realism, it is important to identify structures or mechanisms that, under certain conditions, support actual phenomena and events or cause them to take place (Bhaskar, 2002; Danermark et al., 2003). Therefore, coping practices must be seen with an interdisciplinary approach that focuses on the relation between the individual and the environment, between structure (living reality of the agent) and actor/agent, and these practices must be understood as process-oriented and systemic.

From a CR perspective, the knowledge production with a focus on mechanisms involves taking into account mechanisms on many levels (from molecular, biological, psychological, social and cultural) and describing how mechanisms work on different level of strata in specific situations. In my studies, knowledge about boys' behavioural problems was treated as something more than just biological (Solem, 2013b). Altogether, at different levels, biological, psychological and social mechanisms were in play in the children's situations. In a transitive way, I saw the child's interactional problems in the families with a systemic understanding influencing the behaviour of the boys, but the intransitive explanation could be that neuro-psychological factors from a systemic understanding caused learning problems, hampered boys' interactions with other people and again developed conflicts in interactions. Focus on social factors in a transitive way may see a child's interactional problems in specific social practice. In an intransitive way, a traumatic childhood could be the cause of the interactional problematic situations because emotional problems constructed the interactions that became problematic. This view demands methodological pluralism and respect for other theories and methods in family therapy, where the aim is to develop relevant concepts for the family, linking theory and situated practice together.

CR offered a corrective view, examining parenting phenomena from a comprehensive perspective that considered avoidance strategies as just another part of parents' normal interaction repertoires, and not as causing children's symptoms. All parents have an interaction repertoire, and assess and select suitable actions from this repertoire for particular situations. Avoidance actions and interactions seemed to be different between the two groups. In the comparison group, the parents had resources to withdraw when they were stressed or tired. Some went to a fitness centre to relax, organised their everyday lives with routines and rules so that conflicts with the children were avoided, and had the possibility to hire help, and so on. Some also withdrew from the child from time to time, as some of the parents in clinical group did. Assessed as situated parenting, and not only as generalised strategies, avoidance interactions became a part of the parents' parenting repertoire and were therefore also viewed as proactive interactions.

Family research and CR

Families' socioeconomic situations significantly influenced parenting practices, and may be possibilities or constraints in the caring for their children in the best way possible. It became significant for me to focus on the understanding of parenting practices as situation-specific (quantitatively) and situated (qualitatively). I believe that family research must have practical utility and be useful for families in difficult life situations. This supports the basic tenet that social work research must be value-based. Family research is multidisciplinary, requires a broad understanding and is linked to contexts. Social research may add to clinical social work a broad focus as a supplement to the psychological and health care contributions to practice. It is important have a broad understanding in which knowledge about social inequalities in health is implemented in the knowledge base when professionals meet families in need of help.

In my study, diagnoses are considered as social constructions, but I also see that some children have psychiatric problems. This is in accordance with the concept of double inclusiveness (Bhaskar & Danermark, 2006). My aim was to understand the narrative of the individual parents but to also subsequently look for generating mechanisms for parenting stress and coping practices. These different knowledge types, in this mixed methods study, clarify the picture of telling something important and value-based regarding practice, and to contribute to the scientific basis for professional activities.

The present studies address a gap in our knowledge of parenting by examining and comparing normal family processes, as well as processes in families of children having problems. These studies constructed a model that can be used as a tool in clinical practice to capture living conditions, the organisation of everyday life practices, and child development or family processes together from a child's perspective in assessment of the caring situation.

In clinical practice, knowledge about the "normal" conduct of everyday family life is essential, along with recognition that there must be shifts and breaks in this normalcy, as all family members want to lift themselves out of the ordinariness of everyday life from time to time (Dreier, 2008). Results from research into family relationships can offer clinicians a new understanding of parenthood. CR made me aware of the concepts and discourses of normalcy and diagnosis. It is crucial to study normal family processes because not enough is known about normal coping practices in families. Studying these practices, informed by parents' own reflections, beliefs and framings and organisation of family life from a health-promoting perspective provides important knowledge for family therapy.

Quantitative and qualitative tracks cross each other

Philosophical assumptions guide the data collection and analysis, and the mixture of qualitative and quantitative approaches, in many phases of the research process (Brewer & Hunter, 2006; Creswell & Plano Clark, 2007; Tashakkori & Teddlie, 2003). The methodology chosen depends on what one is trying to do and less on a commitment to a particular paradigm (Cavaye, 1996). The search for complementary and/or confirmatory results is well served by the multi-method research (Creswell et al., 2004). Different models highlight different aspects of a phenomenon or may even constitute different phenomena (Tashakkori & Teddlie, 2003). Qualitative and quantitative methods have traditionally been seen as opposites, as irreconcilable paradigms, because of their different ontological and epistemological positions. However, an increasing number of researchers are saying that this dichotomy is false and outdated (Henningsen & Søndergaard, 2000). By combining both approaches, one may obtain more complementary information about a problem (Brewer & Hunter, 2006; Creswell et al., 2003; Henningsen & Søndergaard, 2000). This is in accordance with CR that favours pluralism, but not relativism. CR was chosen as the metatheory for the current studies because it enabled me to link different theories and perspectives together in the thesis.

Widerberg (2001) argued that both qualitative and quantitative approaches help researchers interpret each other's results. The qualitative study made it possible to go deeper into certain issues to better understand certain unexpected quantitative results, especially when parents' intentions were taken into account. First, I chose both inductive and deductive methodology. Some of the results from the quantitative studies were also used in the qualitative studies. The interpretation of all this data, together with stress and coping theories, may be seen as an abduction process, giving a stronger inference in the data. As a whole, I used sequential exploratory design because it provided stronger inferences. The research process was sequential in the sense that the quantitative analyses were carried out before the qualitative analysis (Creswell & Plano, 2007, Tashakkori & Teddlie, 2003). In such a two-phase design (Creswell, 1994), research first avails itself of a quantitative method to explore patterns in the relationship between the studied phenomena.

I found it important to expand the understanding of parental practices and integrate the understanding of parental coping, by studying parents' meaning making from an everyday life perspective, combined with structural constraints in the parents' environments. From this theoretical standpoint, the integration of quantitative and qualitative methods may be the only way to produce valid and meaningful theoretical explanations in domains in which knowledge of the typical intentions of actors is not immediately available to the researcher (Tashakkori & Teddlie, 2003). The varying perspectives opened up by different methods can supplement each other to produce a more comprehensive picture of the empirical domain under study, which would not be the case if only a single method were applied. Bourdieu and Wacquant (1992) stated that a theory of practice must combine an empathetic and understanding perspective with an explanatory perspective. The causal aims of the present research extended only to the parents' intentions and to exploring patterns of relationships between the phenomena studied as "causal tendencies". I have acknowledged how parents make meaning of their experiences and have also considered how the larger social context impinges on those meanings, while keeping the empirical material and outer limits of "reality" in mind (Braun & Clarke, 2006).

Survey instruments have been followed up with interviews for complementary and confirmatory reasons. In the current case, by combining these approaches, we can see whether the parents' views as captured by the interviews and by the questionnaires either converge or diverge. A researcher will normally choose to interview a few individuals who participated in the survey to learn more about their responses. In the current research, all 192 parents who completed the self-reports were also interviewed. This was done because additional information was needed for use in the quantitative analysis, and because the sensitive nature of the items in the questionnaires made it necessary to meet and interview all parents after they had provided the survey data. The letter accompanying the informed consent statement informed the parents that it was desirable for me (the researcher) to visit them in their homes for an interview after they had completed the self-reports and granted consent. Many parents reported waiting to be called for an interview; because of the sensitive nature of the information, they wanted to meet the person who would handle the information they provided.

Conclusion

It is important to study parenting using a situated approach. Analysis of situated parenting from a developmental perspective in the interviews indicated that parental living conditions affected parent-child interactions, and that these conditions were embedded in the structure of the child's life. This everyday life perspective is a significant analytic tool for clinical social work practice. Social work theories need to go beyond focusing on cultural issues with little emphasis on the individual, and also beyond focusing on intra-psychic issues with minimal attention to the environment (Cornell, 2006). We also know that families exist in constantly changing situations as children and adults grow and develop. However, families' patterns of interaction change slowly and are stable enough to constitute a meaningful research focus (Solem, 2000). It is important to go beyond the simplistic dichotomy of stability versus process – social research projects often tend to analyse phenomena either as stable conditions or as changes or processes. The everyday life of families includes both changes and stability, because family life is framed by organising routines that cannot be repeated exactly. Everywhere in family life we see regularity, habits and routines that enable people to function together without always having to reflect on trivialities and make conscious choices (Dreier, 2008). Routines, the rhythm of activities, and the organising of tasks and habits frame the parenting situation.

These studies reconceptualised parenting stress into situational and relational stress (Solem et al., 2011). Situational stress can be lessened with the help of parent training and similar educational programmes. These offer the potential to improve coping strategies in different contexts and to help parents develop more social support and practical help. Many parents were ashamed of their boys' behaviour and withdrew from friends and family as a result. It is important to be aware of this problem in clinical practice. Relational stress may best be treated through a good working alliance between client and therapist, focused on helping parents manage their children in more effective ways. Other parents may need professional assistance in strengthening their insecure attachment relationships with their children.

Havnen et al., 2009 wrote that researchers have discussed whether interactional problems can be regarded as symptoms or causes of mental health problems. To determine whether interactional problems represent a unique risk factor independent of individual problems constructed by the parent or the child, it is necessary to control for several risk factors associated with the children, the parent and the environment. The concept of parenting stress, as validated in the current research and broken down into the concepts of relational and situational stress may help advance systematic assessments together with investigations of parental resources in family treatment planning and in research.

The current study also challenges the mainstream assumptions about normal family functioning. Knowledge of normal parenting challenges established categories of what constitutes clinical and normal behaviour and cases, with respect to informing clinical practice. The growing diversity and complexity of families makes it imperative to examine the social constructs of normality that powerfully influence all clinical theory and practice, family research and social policy. Therefore, the normal variations regarding family processes will be stretched to include more diversity. In clinical research, it is important to examine the explicit and implicit assumptions about family normality that are embedded in our cultural and clinical belief systems (Walsh, 2003). This includes challenging the stigmatisation of differences as pathological by bringing a clear-eyed understanding of normality back to clinical practice.

References

Archer, M. S. (1995) *Realist Social Theory: The Morphogenetic Approach*, Cambridge: Cambridge University Press.

Bhaskar, R. (2002) *Reflections on Meta-Reality: Transcendence, Emancipation and Everyday Life*, London: Sage.

Bhaskar, R., & Danermark, B. (2006) Metatheory, interdisciplinarity and disability research – A critical realist perspective, *Scandinavian Journal of Disability Research*, 4, 278–297.

Bourdieu, P., & Wacquant, L. J. D. (1992) *An Invitation to Reflexive Sociology*, Chicago, IL: University of Chicago Press.

Braun, V., & Clarke, V. (2006) Using thematic analysis in psychology, *Qualitative Research in Psychology*, 3, 77–101.

Brewer, J., & Hunter, A. (2006) A Postscript on Postmodernism. In Brewer, J. & Hunter, A. (eds.), *Foundations of Multimethod Research: Synthesizing Styles*, Thousand Oaks, CA: Sage, pp. 151–162.

Cavaye, A. L. M. (1996) Case study research: A multi-faceted research approach for IS, *Information Systems Journal*, 6, 227–242.

Collins, K. M. T., Onwuegbuzie, A. J., & Jiao, Q. G. (2010) *Toward a Broader Understanding of Stress and Coping: Mixed Methods Approaches*, Charlotte, NC: Information Age Publishing.

Cornell, K. L. (2006) Person-in-situation: History, theory, and new directions for social work practice, *Praxis*, 6, 50–57.

Creswell, J. W. (1994) *Research Design: Qualitative and Quantitative Approaches*, Thousand Oaks, CA: Sage.

Creswell, J. W., Fetters, M. D., & Ivankova, N. V. (2004) Designing a mixed methods study in primary care, *Annuals of Family Medicine*, 32, 7–12.

Creswell, J. W., & Plano Clark, V. L. (2007) *Designing and Conducting Mixed Methods Research*, Thousand Oaks, CA: Sage.

Creswell, J. W., Plano Clark, V. L., Gutmann, M. L., & Hanson, W. E. (2003) Advanced Mixed Methods Research Designs. In Tashakkori, A. & Teddlie, C. (eds.), *Handbook of Mixed Methods in Social and Behavioural Research*, Thousand Oaks, CA: Sage, pp. 209–240.

Danermark, B., Ekström, M., Jakobsen, L., & Karlsson, J. C. (2003) *Att forklara samhället. [To Explain Society]*, Lund: Studentlitteratur AB.

Dreier, O. (2008) *Psychotherapy in Everyday Life*, Cambridge: Cambridge University Press.

Havnen, K. S., Jakobsen, R., & Stormark, K. M. (2009) Mental health problems in Norwegian school children placed out-of-home: The importance of family risk factors, *Child Care in Practice*, 15, 235–250.

Henningsen, I., & Søndergaard, D. M. (2000) Forskningstradisjoner krydser deres spor. Kvalitative og kvantitative socio-kulturelle empiriske forskningsmetoder [Research traditions crossing tracks: Qualitative and quantitative socio – Cultural empirical research methods], *Kvinder, Køn & Forskning*, 4, 26–38.

Lloyd, T., & Hastings, R. P. (2008) Psychological variables as correlates of adjustment in mothers of children with intellectual disabilities: Cross-sectional and longitudinal relationships, *Journal of Intellectual Disability Research*, 52(1), 37–48.

Rogoff, B. (1990) *Apprenticeship in Thinking: Cognitive Development in Social Context*, New York: Oxford University Press.

Rogoff, B. (1997) Evaluating Development in the Process of Participation: Theory, Methods, and Practice Building on Each Other. In Amsel, E. & Renninger, A. (eds.), *Change and Development*, Hillsdale, NJ: Lawrence Erlbaum, pp. 679–744.

Sayer, A. (2010) *Method in Social Science: A Realist Approach*, Oxon: Routledge.

Solem, M. B. (2000) Å ta empirien med en klype salt: Sentrale problemer i familieforskning I barne- og ungdomspsykiatrien. Del 1: Målemetodenes reliabilitet og validitet [Empirism taken with a pinch of salt: Significant problems in family research in child and adolescent psychiatry: Reliability and validity of family measurement techniques], *Fokus på familien*, 4, 254–264.

Solem, M. B. (2011) *Parenting Stress and Coping Practices: A Salutogenic Approach*, Oslo: Department of Psychology, Faculty of Social Sciences, University of Oslo.

Solem, M. B. (2013a) Meaning making and avoidance in parenting, *Qualitative Social Work*, 12, 170–185.

Solem, M. B. (2013b) Understanding parenting as situated in the larger sociocultural context: Child in clinical social work, *Child Adolescent Social Work Journal*, 30, 61–78.

Solem, M. B., Christophersen, K. A., & Martinussen, M. (2011) Predicting parenting stress: Children's behavioral problems and parents' coping, *Infant and Child Development*, 20, 162–180.

Tashakkori, A., & Teddlie, C. (2003) *Handbook on Mixed Methods in the Behavioural and Social Sciences*, Thousand Oaks, CA: Sage.

Walsh, F. (2003) *Normal Family Processes: Growing Diversity and Complexity*, New York: Guilford Press.

Widerberg, K. (2001) *Historien om et kvalitativt forskningsprosjekt [Story of a Qualitative Research Project]*, Oslo: Universitetsforlaget.

9   Positions of young people in child welfare

"TMSA" in research practice

Elina Pekkarinen

Introduction

P: I was at home and then my mom said that "today you're not going anywhere; today you're staying at home". I was a bit puzzled about what was going on; why did I have to stay at home? Who was coming, and what was going on? I stayed at home, however, and then the doorbell rang. And there were these two women waiting outside and they told me that "This is it, this is the thing; you're coming with us".

(Interview)[1]

The above citation is part of an interview in which a 24-year-old former reform school student describes how he was placed in out-of-home care by child welfare at the age of 12. He had grown up with a single mother, four siblings, and a step-father, who used disciplinary violence toward the children. Prior to the placement, he had a period of increasing conflicts at home. He did not obey the rules set by the parents, skipped school, used alcohol, and hung around with peers of the same neighbourhood, drifting into petty crimes and other disruptive behaviour. When being told to pack his backpack by the social workers, he had never heard of child welfare, foster care, or reform schools. The incident at the home door was the beginning of a period in life that took him to five different institutions in six years. During these years, he experienced neglect and powerlessness, but also support and emancipation. Now, years later, he wants to make sure that this does not happen to other children in similar circumstances.

The reader might think that the incident took place decades ago. However, when this 12-year-old was being taken out of his house by two strangers, with no explanation of what was going on, it was the beginning of a new millennium in a middle-size city in the Nordic welfare state of Finland. Since the 1980s, children in Finland have had a strong legal position in child welfare. As early as 1983, it was stated in the Finnish Child Welfare Act that children's opinions – regardless of their chronological age – had to be clarified and taken into account in the decision-making process. In 2007, children that were 12 years of age and older were given an internationally exceptional right to speak for themselves in child welfare proceedings, including in the court, if court proceedings were involved. Thus, a child age 12 years or older may demand his care order to be overturned, he has a right to appeal, and a right to demand child welfare services (Pösö & Huhtanen, 2016). However, the practices of child welfare may differ from what the letter of the law presupposes.

Critical realism, and particularly Bhaskar's Transformational Model of Social Activity (TMSA), forms the metatheoretical framework of this empirical piece of text. It describes how the application of TMSA functions as a metatheoretical framework in empirical social work research that applies theoretical concepts from the theory of labelling. It focuses on how Bhaskar's way of perceiving social reality can open windows to individuals' world of experiences, and how individuals' experiences of their own positions, formed in the interaction with others, help to understand the outcomes of these positions in the self-understanding of people who have grown up in threatening circumstances. It reveals how the reactions of others may affect people's understanding of themselves, cause insecurity, difficulties in trusting others, and strengthen their occupancy of the marginal positions. However, it also reveals how the outcomes of these positions are resisted, how alternative identities are constructed, and how the agency of the ones positioned may cause emancipation and transformation of the oppressive social structures. Thus, the article concludes by discussing the role of the past in relation to the present not only in the forms of social structures but in the forms of people's positions and identities as well.

Research questions and theoretical framework of the study

Research questions

In my previous research projects (Pekkarinen, 2010; 2014), I have aimed to find out which mediators (Archer, 1998, p. 372) set off the process of social exclusion. I have been particularly interested in the role of different positions, surrounding agents, and institutions in the process of exclusion, and in what kinds of impact the reactions of other people, and particularly institutional social welfare interventions, have on the individual. In my research I have applied Roy Bhaskar's Transformational Model of Social Activity (TMSA) (1979, pp. 43–47; 1986, pp. 118–136) and the theoretical concepts derived from the theory of societal reaction by Edwin M. Lemert (1951; 1967) to study cases in which child welfare has intervened in young people's lives. With the help of Bhaskar's TMSA, I have created a model which I call *the position model* with which I aim to tame the ambiguous concept of position used by Bhaskar in his TMSA. In this article, I study the application of the model to a qualitative study – in-depth interviews outlining the experiences of eight young adults that have been placed into out-of-home care and finally to reform schools by child welfare agency due to their disruptive and norm-breaking behaviour.

In my research, I have studied how intervention into the situation of children at risk of exclusion takes place and what kinds of impacts the reactions of others have in the children's social relationships and self-perception. When researching the reactions of the surrounding community, I have been interested in child welfare services, as the contradiction between the social control and support that is typical in child welfare is very perceptible. This contradiction is particularly strong in situations in which the freedom of the autonomic agent – usually a teenage child in the cases that I studied – is restricted. My research projects are also related to the field of youth research. I am therefore studying a stage of life which is characterised by the conflict caused by the simultaneous increase in independence and growing social control. Young people have always, in one way or another, been singled out by communities. In this article, I examine the personal experiences of the subjects of the child welfare intervention and how their positions are affected by the dynamic relations of their own agency and the surrounding agents and institutions. I aim to reveal the kind of positions that young people who have been involved with child welfare are being positioned in by the social contexts and different agents they have been involved with; how the young people themselves experience these positions; and how these positions have affected the young people's senses of agency and self-understanding. By this reflection, I aim to find out the role of different positions in a dynamic interplay of relations in these children's external and inner life-worlds.

The position-practice system by Roy Bhaskar

The ultimate target of my research is to demonstrate how the children's positions are affected by institutional and societal structures, agents, societal reactions and the child's own agency, and how the children themselves experience these positions. With the help of empirical data, I will apply the model to which I have incorporated elements based on Bhaskar's TMSA and on Edwin M. Lemert's theory of societal reactions. Particularly interesting in Bhaskar's TMSA is the position-practice system, which he argues is a system of mediating concepts that comprises the 'point of contact' in which agents meet the social structures (1979, pp. 51–52; 1986, pp. 130–131; 1993, p. 156). However, Bhaskar is not precise with his definition of the position-practice system, an issue that Margaret Archer has taken on, and argued to a great extent (1995; 1998; 2000). This vagueness of defining is not solely an issue with the concept of the position-practice system, but other central concepts as well. For example, in Bhaskar's TMSA, the definition of social structure has often been under debate (see e.g. Porpora, 1998; Archer, 1998; Kaidesoja, 2009). However, Bhaskar is not the only philosopher in the history of social sciences to have problems in defining social structures. Douglas V. Porpora argues that in spite of social structure being one of the most central concepts in sociology, there is wide disagreement on what it means (Porpora, 1998, p. 339). Porpora himself identifies four prominent alternative conceptions of social structure: 1) social structures as patterns of aggregate behaviour; 2) as a system of law-like regularities among social facts; 3) as systems of human relations among social positions; and 4) as rules and resources (Porpora, 1993). He locates critical realists to the third conception – understanding social structure as systems of human relations among social positions – and Bhaskar verifies this conclusion in many of his texts.

According to Bhaskar, society does not consist of individuals, but expresses *the sum of the relations* within which individuals stand (Bhaskar, 1979, p. 32). Before identifying social structure as systems of human relations among social positions, however, one has to define the concepts of human relations and that of social position. Bhaskar states that because social structures are continually reproduced and are exercised only in human agency, a *system of mediating concepts* is needed for comprising this "point of contact" or "slots" in which agents meet the structures.

> Such a point, linking action to structure, must *both* endure and be immediately occupied by individuals. It is clear that the mediating system we need is that of the *positions* (places, functions, rules, tasks, duties, rights, etc.) occupied (filled, assumed, enacted) by individuals, and of the *practices* (activities, etc.) in which, in virtue of their occupancy of these positions (and vice-versa), they engage. I shall call this mediating system the position-practice system. Now such positions and practices, if they are to be individuated at all, can only be done so *relationally*.
>
> (Bhaskar, 1998, pp. 40–41)

Thus, according to Bhaskar, these positions are structurally constituted, and even though they are occupied by individuals, they cannot ontologically be reduced to the occupation of individual agents. According to Bhaskar, the relations can neither be reduced only to interpersonal relations, but to relations with nature and social products too, and that the relations must be conceptualised holding between the positions and practices – not between individual agents (Bhaskar, 1998, p. 41).

These positions and the relations among social positions (e.g. social structures) are the central theoretical concepts of this research. Even though Bhaskar's philosophical realism can be described as a "general platform, capable of underpinning various social theories", and his TMSA as a "social theory in its own right" (Archer, 1998, p. 357), it does not provide concepts for explaining the phenomena I am interested in. I have a theoretical assumption that the social structures within this position-practice system produce mechanisms or mediators that cause processes with certain outcomes, and that these outcomes may transform the positions as well. Through the societal reaction theory, I have found theoretical concepts for describing how these positions are occupied by the agents, what intended and unintended consequences may derive others' reactions to these positions, and how people's identities are affected by the social positions they occupy.

The theory of societal reaction

The theory of societal reaction has its roots in the Neo-Chicago School, which is based on, for example, the symbolic interactionism of Charles Horton Cooley (1864–1929) and George Herbert Mead (1863–1931). Labelling theories begin with the assumption that *no act is intrinsically abnormal* because *deviance only arises from the imposition of social judgements on others' behaviour.* These judgements are established, maintained, formulated, and interpreted by societies' agents, and especially by the powerful – the legislators, police, courts, and other controlling institutions, such as social work (Muncie, 2004, pp. 117–122; Garland, 2001, pp. 65–66; Lemert, 2000c, pp. 71–72; Petrunik, 1980; Taylor et al., 1973, pp. 139–141). The core of these theories is at the processes these judgements may trigger. At its simplest, these theorists suggest that "the attempt to deter, punish and prevent deviation can actually create deviation itself" (Taylor et al., 1973, p. 140). Thus, the labelling theories relate to social constructionist schools of thinking, but one of their theorists – Edwin M. Lemert (1912–1996) – opposed this connection to social constructionism (Lemert, 1974).

Lemert attempted to systemise the study of deviance in terms of social differentiation and social control, and "to discover the circumstances under which the latter gives meaning and shape and stability to socially-evaluated differences of individuals and groups" (Lemert, 2000c, p. 72). Lemert preferred to call his theory one of *societal reaction*, because he was critical of labelling theorists' and interactionists' tendency to forget the contexts in which social interaction takes place (see e.g. Lemert, 1948; Lemert & Winter, 2000). Societal reaction is a concept which directs attention *to the social response to the original act* (Lemert & Winter, 2000, p. 280; Goffman, 1963; Lemert, 1951, pp. 76–77). According to Lemert, the concepts of normal and deviant behaviour vary between cultures and historical periods, and are thus socially constructed to some extent. However, he highlights the genetic, physiological, and objectively observable aspects of deviation. He divides the aspects of deviation to overt and covert, overt referring to visibly deviant behaviour and covert deviance referring to something not directly observed, such as attitudes and emotions (Lemert, 1951, pp. 34–36). Thus, we should consider the individual, situational, and systematic functions when approaching deviance. One significant social factor related to deviance is that of societal reaction (Ibid., pp. 37–44, 54).

For Lemert, the concept of societal reaction is a very general term, which summarises both the expressive reactions of others and the actions directed at controlling deviance. In his writings, Lemert was particularly interested in the position of young offenders in the control agencies. He was a strong opponent of youth courts due to their stigmatising nature, and emphasised the multifaceted problems in young offenders' lives (Lemert & Winter, 2000, pp. 198–216; Lemert, 1951, pp. 304–305). The essential message of Lemert's theory was that *the reactions of the surrounding social system have an impact on a child's identity development, and should not include potentially stigmatising aspects.* Lemert justified this conclusion with his concepts of primary and secondary deviation. These concepts underpin the essential effect of societal reaction to the development of internalised deviancy, and motivate us to study the responses we direct at others. According to Lemert:

> the deviations remain primary deviations or symptomatic and situational as long as they are rationalised or otherwise dealt with as functions of a socially

acceptable role. *When a person begins to employ his deviant behavior or a role based upon it as a means of defense, attack, or adjustment to the overt or covert problems created by the consequent societal reaction to him, his deviation is secondary.*

(Lemert, 1951, pp. 75–76)

According to Lemert, the sequence of interactions that lead to secondary deviance are dynamic and individual in a sense that people's characteristic traits and their capacity to cope with others' reactions vary. This dynamic process takes place in a structured context – within sets of external and internal limits. With external limits, Lemert refers to those constructed by society in the form of barriers to social participation. In addition to these external limits are the subjective components of human personality, which he calls the internal limits. There is continuous interplay between external and internal limits, and this interrelationship has an impact on the selection of the social positions available for an individual (Lemert, 1951, pp. 81–85). A person's adjustment to different positions depends on the congruence between the societal definition and the individual's self-understanding. A person may adjust, interjecting the societal definition as his self-understanding and playing the associated position – or he may resist it. There are also situations where the societal positions differ from a person's self-understanding so radically that no alternatives are open to the individual. This conflict can lead to total destruction of the individual's mind (ibid., pp. 91–95).

Merging Bhaskar's position-practice system with Lemert's theory of societal reaction

My understanding of social reality consists of the plane of agency (i.e. agents and praxis of the social context) and the plane of structure (i.e. structural elements of the social context). Neither plane is existent without the other or by itself sufficient for understanding the social conditions of existence and human activity. When defining a position of an individual, these planes are connected by two dimensions – *the individual's external and inner life-worlds* (*Lebenswelt,* see Bhaskar, 1986, p. 128). These planes and dimensions are demonstrated in Figure 9.1 and explained in more detail next.

In this model, the individual's external life-world has two domains – the external conditions and external definitions of action. By *external conditions of action,* I refer to those conditions that affect our social participation and are dimensions of social structures (Bhaskar, 1979, p. 47). At times, these conditions may form what Lemert has called *external limits* – barriers to social participation arising from the social and cultural environment. Examples of external limits are those based on age, sex, physical characteristics, economic status, geographic and demographic factors, and mobility (Lemert, 1951, pp. 82–85), but these limits may go beyond these measurable traits, such as cultural norms and values. It is also important to state that the external conditions should not be studied only from the limiting viewpoint, as they may also be the structural requisites that enable social action.

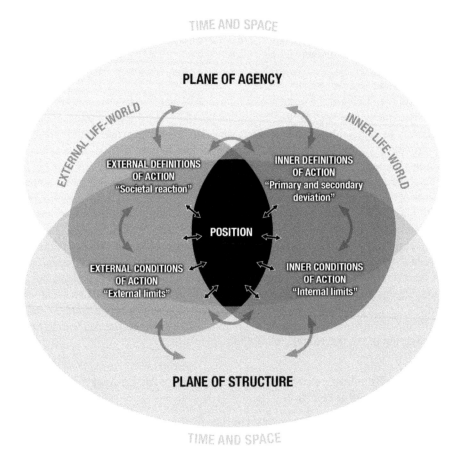

Figure 9.1 The system of agency, structure, individual's life-world, and position

By *external definitions of the individual's action,* I refer to the responses of people and societal agents to the individual's actions. These are what Lemert calls *societal reactions,* and they form the conceptual base of his theory (Lemert, 1951, p. 449). These reactions depend not only on the action and actor itself but also on the position the individual is occupying, and the historical and cultural dimensions this positions carries. The societal reactions may be informal expressive reactions and attitudes that may carry emotional dimensions and that are witnessed in the everyday relations of individuals or groups. Informal societal reactions may also be extended and formalised to institutional agencies that are given the responsibility to carry out practices that are connected to these formalised positions (Lemert & Winter, 2000, pp. 31–32). Child welfare practices are an example of institutionalised and formalised societal reactions.

Just as the individual's external life-world, the inner life-world has two domains as well – the inner conditions and inner definitions of action. By *inner conditions of action,* I refer to what Lemert has called the *internal limits* – the attitudes, knowledge, skills, and experiences – of personality, which may restrict or enlarge the choice-making of the individual (Lemert, 1951, p. 87, 448). Bhaskar's model of the interplay of social conditions, praxis and the individual's inner capabilities is almost identical to Lemert's notion of internal limits:

> unintended consequences and unacknowledged conditions may limit the actors' understanding of their social world, while unacknowledged (unconscious) motivation and tacit skills may limit his or her understanding of him or herself.
> (Bhaskar, 1986, p. 126)

By *inner definitions of action,* I refer to Lemert's concepts of *primary and secondary deviation*, which were defined in detail earlier. Societal reactions may or may not have an impact on the individual's sense of self. As long as the individual can exclude the labels as not attached to his self-understanding, his deviance is primary. However, the moment the individual begins to accept the definitions of others as part of his self-understanding, his identity – and often agency – begins to change. Sometimes this new identity carries a negative stigma, sometimes it may work as an emancipating tool. In reference to emancipation, Bhaskar (1986) discusses the possibility of false consciousness and individuals' opportunities to become aware of these internalised definitions – often derived from the external definitions. This is exactly the reason I claim that taking the individual's own perceptions of positions into account is important, despite the critical realist notion of position being an objective phenomenon independent of individual occupancy. In real life, positions are usually individuated and to understand the effects of being positioned in a certain way – by other people, institutions, or one's own false or real perception – it is important to be able to intervene in the social processes followed by these positions in the cases where the outcomes are negative for individuals or groups. Understanding both – external and inner – dimensions of the position enables a true transformation in the social structures that relate these domains to one another.

As these dimensions – external and internal conditions and definitions of action – form a dynamic interplay between individuals and groups, and as the relations between these relations (see Bhaskar, 1979, p. 36) in time and place occur, different *positionings* take place, and different *positions* are created and reconstructed. The arrows in Figure 9.1 represent the inner social structure of the position – the causal properties such as tendencies, forces, and capabilities of the position formed by the relations in between the different domains (see Porpora, 1998, p. 343). Thus, I define a position as a point of convergence of agency and structure, which is affected by the dynamic interplay and relations between the individual's or group's inner and external conditions and definitions of action in a social context situated in time and space.

This definition of position is more flexible and affected by subjective actions than the traditional definition of a position as a "passive aspect of role" (see Archer, 1998, pp. 371–372). At the same time, this definition of position is more structural, compared with the use of the concepts by positioning theorists such as Rom Harré and Luk van Langenhove (Harré & Langenhove, 1999) that define potential positions as being dependent on how one can use discourses, and as "a cluster of short-term disputable rights, obligations and duties" (Harré, 2012, p. 193). By referring to Bhaskar's philosophy inspired by Marx, I think that a person seldom has the opportunity to negotiate his positions, when facing interaction in the structured and institutionalised social world we live in. He has, however, the possibility of interpreting and analysing the effects of these positions through his own experiences – and thus of trying to intervene in the social and personal consequences of these positions.

Data and method

In my previous research, I have applied the position model in case studies analysing the interventions of child welfare through document data (Pekkarinen, 2010; 2014). However, analysis of document data does not give an insight into how young people themselves experience the child welfare interventions, and the positions they occupy. In my postdoctoral research,[2] I wanted to find out how children who had been placed into out-of-home care, due to their disruptive behaviour, experienced these interventions and their positions. In order to get in touch with these young people, I participated in a development group formed by former students of Finnish reform schools[3] for two years in 2014 and 2015, and carried phenomenological in-depth interviews (Seidman, 2013) with eight of these young adults.

In this article, I call the interviewees participants to reflect their active stance in the interviews (Seidman, 2013, p. 14). Six of the participants were women and two were men, and they were between 22 and 28 years old. The interviews were carried out in locations chosen by the participants, and lasted approximately two hours each. The framework of the interviews was based on asking the participants to describe their life prior to the child welfare interventions, why and how child welfare was involved in their lives, and their experiences of the first and following placements to out-of-home care. I also asked the participants to describe how and why they were placed in reform school, their experiences of reform school, and what happened afterward. At the end of the interviews, I asked the participants to reflect on the significance of the child welfare interventions in relation to their current situations and future. The interviews were recorded and transcribed, and the transcriptions were analysed by ATLAS.ti software for qualitative data analysis. The data was coded within 10 thematic code-families, which concluded into 189 codes that were attached to 679 parts of the data over 3,000 times. One could call the analysis of the data "thick coding", and it made visible the different institutional structures and situations, and different agents, emotions, and feelings attached to different experiences in life. Through the analysis, I focused my viewpoint on the positions of these young people in different phases of their lives, and to the meanings of the experiences that these positions raised in them.

Carrying out the interviews has required intensive ethical considerations, and the ethical guidelines of the Finnish Advisory Board for Research Integrity were carefully followed. The participants signed a written consent and were given the opportunity to withdraw from the study. The research articles written in Finnish were given to the participants for comments before their publication. In order to anonymize the participants, I have not used individuated numbers in the citations of the interviews, and I have neutralized their sexes by using s/he, hem, and hir instead of she or he, him or her, and his or her. I have also changed some details, and avoided using the parts of the interviews that might lead to the identification of the people involved. The issues that were handled in the interviews were extremely sensitive and brought difficult memories for the participants, so I encouraged them to contact counselling if they felt they needed to reflect upon some of the issues that were brought up. I also gave them the opportunity to keep in touch with me, and some of the participants have continued to do so.

Both the data and the subject of this article could be characterized as extreme. Taking a child into care, and placing him or her into out-of-home care, is an exceptional intervention, and particularly reform schools are places which take in the most demanding groups of young people. In this article, only the viewpoint of the young people is being described, and this reveals only one side of the reality. It is important to keep these features of the data in mind while reading the following chapters.

Positions and experiences of young people on child welfare interventions

Being vulnerable and different: the positions of early childhood

Each of the eight young people who were interviewed had their own personal life story to tell. Behind each of the stories were difficult experiences in early childhood, which were associated with conflicts within the family. Some had experienced parents' substance abuse and mental health problems, domestic violence, sexual abuse, frequently moving house, or neglect. In the following citation, a participant describes hir first experience with the child welfare agency.

P: [–] At that time I was six years old, I think. It began, well, I don't remember too much of that, but I remember us leaving our house in the middle of the night. The leading social worker of [the city] carried my little sister out of our house, because my mother and her current boyfriend got caught. They were dealing drugs back at the end of the '90s, and, well, my mother was sentenced to jail and we had to move to my dad's place.

(Interview)

Five of the participants had had contact with child welfare since very early childhood. Some of them had been placed in out-of-home care either for short periods or permanently, and even the ones who had not been involved with child welfare had contacts with health care or school counselling. When analysing the positions of these children through the societal reactions of others, one could describe these children as vulnerable, a concept that represents the experiences of the participants as well. Even though the difficult situations of these children were noticed by the surrounding communities, it was common for the needs of the children to be overshadowed by the difficulties of the adults. Being vulnerable and not receiving adequate help caused insecurity and difficulties in trusting other people.

One of the participants described, how hir father's heavy drinking and violent behaviour continuously forced the family to move to a secure shelter, and how the feelings of insecurity made it difficult for hem to focus on anything other than worrying about hir mother's well-being. The vulnerable position of the participant is described in Figure 9.2, where the basic structure and context

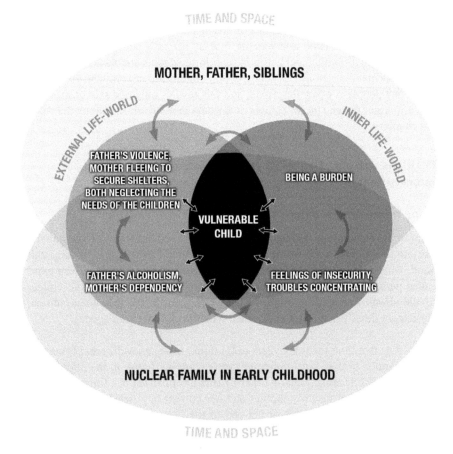

Figure 9.2 The position of a vulnerable child in the system of structure, agency, and individual's life-world

of the position is placed in a nuclear family with external conditions defined by the father's alcoholism, and the mother's inability to separate from the abusive relationship. The actions taken by the surrounding adults are defined by the father's violence, and by the mother escaping the house with the children. None of the adults were able to take care of the needs of the children. In these circumstances, the child's experiences of hir vulnerable position result in feelings of insecurity and inability to concentrate on issues that could be regarded as typical for a normal child. This participant had a strong sense of being a burden to the family.

Even in the mildest cases, feelings of being a burden to the guardians were common. These experiences were connected with feelings of being different among peers. Six of the participants explained that they had felt different since childhood, because of either their behaviour or looks, and had been singled out because of this in various everyday communities. Sometimes the feeling of being different was strengthened by severe bullying.

> I was in the canteen and remember that everyone was white, absolutely everyone was white (–). And I dropped my milk on the floor there in the canteen, and one boy started bashing the table like this and was like 'lick it up, lick it up and you'll become white, lick it up, lick it up, you'll become white' (bashes the table) and everyone laughed! Not one teacher, not one person did a thing and they all saw.
>
> *(Interview)*

When analysed within the framework of the position model, in addition to being vulnerable, one could define the positions of these children among their peers and everyday communities as one of being different. This position of being different was experienced by the participants as being an outsider, feeling lonely, and being bullied, not only by the other children but by adults as well. Most traumatizing had been the cases in which the person responsible for the bullying was in a position of authority to the child, such as a guardian or a teacher. School was often the context in which bullying took place, just as in the previous citation. Only two participants had been diagnosed with learning difficulties, but all of them shared experiences of having severe difficulties at school, and not being either able or motivated to follow the teaching. In the following section, the participants' positions in early adolescence are being described.

From vulnerable to defiant: the positions of early adolescence

Despite the severe difficulties at home, the majority of the participants continued to live with their parents. Often the family was reduced to being a one-parent family, if the other parent ever had been present. As they became older, all of the participants ended up in conflict at home with their siblings and guardians. The problems did not stay within the home walls either. Instead, conflicts at school with teachers and often with other pupils were followed by loafing in the streets, and breaking the rules both at home and in the neighbourhood. Some of the young people used intoxicants and committed crimes – but not all of them. Disruptive behaviour was sometimes targeted to the self, and three of the participants had seriously injured themselves before finally being taken into care. By the time the intervention took place, a position of a defiant, difficult, and at times even a dangerous youth was the position held for the participants. This position was followed by interventions, which were implemented with speed and force and that gave no room for negotiation and change. Being placed into out-of-home care came as a shock for the majority of the participants. In the following citation, one participant describes how s/he had to be cheated into going to a psychiatric ward for children after being suspended from school.

P: [–] The situation was such that during that so-called summer vacation, I didn't do anything sensible. And after that being taken into care was the next station. And that next place was a psychiatric ward for children in [our city].

E: And that happened after the fifth grade?

P: Yeah.

E: Okay. Can you recall any of the conversations prior to the hospital?

P: Nobody had any conversations with me.

E: Okay, so they didn't have conversations with you. Did they tell you that this placement would happen?

P: No. They had to cheat me into it.

E: Oh no.

P: Oh yeah. My stepmother said, "let's go and see your new school. We'll just go and have a look". Off we went, and then she said, "be polite, and go through the door first", and the door closed behind me.

E: Unbelievable. [P: Mm-m]. Didn't she even walk you in there?

P: No, she turned away at the door.

(Interview)

This participant had already spent hir early childhood in a children's home, and eight years in a foster family. After running into trouble at school, s/he was suspended, and finally taken into a hospital. S/he cannot remember anyone telling hem about the plan to place hem into a hospital for one-and-a-half years. Instead, s/he was cheated there by hir stepmother. Not being told what was going to happen was repeated in all the major turns of hir early life. In the later part of the interview, s/he stated that 99 percent of hir problems in life were due to the fact that in different phases of hir life s/he was never told or given a precise explanation of why s/he was treated as s/he was. The door that closed behind hir back was the beginning of a period in different institutions that continued until the participant was 21 years old. This experience of being ignored, not knowing their own rights, lack of influence and uncertainty was common to all of the participants.

This was a continuation of the insecurity experienced in early childhood, and now the young people reacted by acting out.

P: I was involved in this [pauses]. Well it was this one thing that took place outside the school. I had these really bad fights with this one [young person], and then it sort of got totally out of hand. There were some friends of mine, and we had an argument with this [person] again, and then one of my friends went to hir house. And hir mother was at home, and this friend of mine smashed their windows in with a baseball bat. Like totally smashed them into millions of pieces.

(Interview)

The position of a defiant problem youth was thus strengthened by the young people's own behaviour. They described how the position was experienced by them as legitimising their disruptive behaviour. In Lemert's concepts, one could state that the position had an effect on their deviance becoming secondary – an internalised part of their self-understanding (ibid., 1951, p. 76). Thus, the position of a defiant was deepened by a process where both the external and internal mechanisms and mediators pushed their exclusion further, and caused both external and internalised labelling and stigmatization. Figure 9.3 illustrates how the position of a defiant problem youth was formed in the dynamic of external and internal conditions and definitions.

Being in care: the position of a reform school student

All of the participants were eventually taken into out-of-home care by the child welfare agency, but for most of them, the road to the reform school was winding and had many placements before the final destination of reform school. The feeling of being excluded, ignored, and having a lack of influence followed them all the way. Some of them experienced abuse and neglect in foster families, children's homes or youth shelters prior to the reform school placement. Lack of supervision in Finnish foster families and child welfare institutions has constantly been the focus of public debate. For the participants, the lack of supervision was one part of the problem, but even more severe were the situations where their stories were not taken seriously. In the following citation, the participant had been placed in an institution that practiced isolation orders that were not in line with Finnish legislation. The young people were accompanied by an adult at all times, they were not allowed to have unsupervised phone calls with their parents, and using their native language was forbidden. Also slightly less humiliating incidents, such as having a birthday cake baked for them, and not being allowed to eat it, took place. When the participant told hir social worker of these practices, the carers were present at the meeting, and denied hir stories.

E: How did if feel when they didn't believe you?

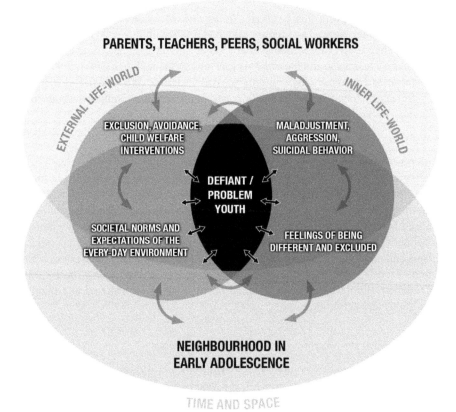

Figure 9.3 The position of a defiant/problem youth in the system of structure, agency, and individual's life-world

P: It felt really wrong, really wrong. I was trying to tell it like I saw it, of course, and the experiences of young people – they are not taken seriously. They always underestimate you and of course young people feel things differently. So they think that you exaggerate things, and they look at you like "what are you babbling on about again". But it's not like that. It's not always like that [long pause].

(Interview)

Being placed in a reform school was the final stop for all but one of the participants. Reform schools have a reputation for being institutions with strict discipline and dangerous delinquents, so placement felt scary for most of them. One of the participants described how s/he stayed awake for the first night and was convinced s/he would die. Another became a target of serious bullying again, and felt s/he was not being listened to about hir suffering. Another one became distanced from all the other students and concentrated on hir studies. However, at the time of the interview, they all felt that the placement in the reform school was a relief and a turning point in their lives.

P: Well, if the things would've gone differently, if I had not been taken into care and had not been placed in the [reform school], I very likely wouldn't be alive anymore. My behaviour was so suicidal that it would had been very likely that I would have died, or at least been in a very bad shape.

E: What do you think was the most important thing that affected this situation being as it is now?

P: Maybe [thinks for a while]. Well maybe when I was doing these stupid things before, I felt that I was, I dunno, somehow bad or something. I felt I couldn't do anything and wasn't good at anything. I felt like I was worth nothing. But then there, it began, I started to feel better, and I started to really understand, because you were encouraged to do it, you were told that "hey, you know how to do it; you're really good at this and that, so why don't you try this too". And then I realized that I'm not stupid. I've been lost, but I'm not stupid. And it started to have an effect on me. I felt that I found a light in me, and I began to feel that I wanna do wise stuff, and not just hang around out there.

(Interview)

Being encouraged and trusted gave this participant a strong sense of emancipation, and a feeling that s/he could learn and succeed in life. These feelings of being saved or being woken up were common to all the participants. This contradiction – being placed in an institution with a reputation for having the most challenging and dangerous residents, and at the same time having an experience of finding a new road in life – was distinctive to the position of a reform school student. The prejudices of other people and the societal reactions following them were noticed by the participants themselves.

P: There was this elementary school and a sports track just next to it. And once we went there as a group, you know we went jogging, and then there were these elementary school students out there, and you know what they said? They were like, "eeeww, the criminals are there, stay away, don't go there, I mean it, don't go, they're the students from the [reform school], they are like true gangstas, totally messed up!" We had like this sign over here [points at her forehead] that said [the name of the reform school]. Everybody knew who we were, and they immediately thought we were messed up – that we were crazy, that we were bad people, and if you're a bad person or you have problems in your head, you're placed there. I mean, they threaten and scare children by saying that if you don't obey the rules; you will be taken into a reform school.

(Interview)

In the previous description one can see how the other children and adults in the surrounding community reacted to the position of a reform school student. Interestingly, this reputation is common not solely among people who do not know the details of the Finnish reform school system, but also among child welfare professionals: according to the managers of reform schools, the negative attitudes of child welfare professionals postpone placements to reform schools, even though the placement is regarded as being in the best interests of the child (Pekkarinen, 2017). These societal reactions caused insecurity and shame, which is illustrated in Figure 9.4.

Living the label: the position of a former reform school student

Reform school students' negative reputation had far-reaching consequences. Being placed in a reform school intensified the feeling of being different, and the

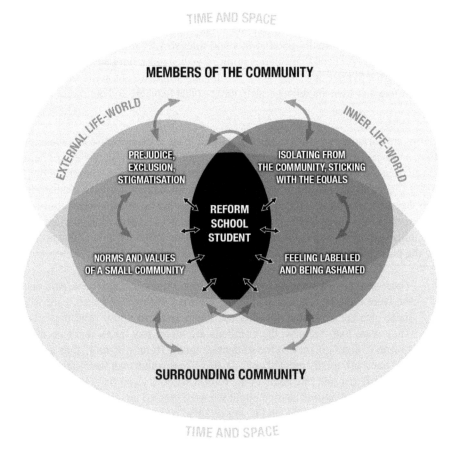

Figure 9.4 The position of a reform school student in the system of structure, agency, and individual's life-world

reputation gained from being in a reform school was felt to have an impact on self-understanding. The experience of being different followed the individual into subsequent environments in the form of reputation. The following participant was placed in an institution closer to home after being in reform school.

P: They [instructors] made the mistake of warning the other young people not to have anything to do with me as I was from a reform school, which meant I was bad. They weren't allowed to have anything to do with me [–]. So then I naturally got carried away, because I was the boss. So you think reform school kids are this bad, well I'll show ya. I have seen what they are like. And I really went for it.

(Interview)

In the previous quotation, the participant started to consciously live the deviant role that had been constructed for hem by the community. According to Lemert's concepts, hir deviance became secondary because of the pressure of the environment – adopted as a result of the environment's reaction, and guiding hir own behaviour and life choices (Lemert, 1951, pp. 75–76). As stated earlier, it was a "mistake" for the instructors to tell others about hir background, and silencing the past had been a coping mechanism for many of the participants. Only one of the participants explained that s/he had always been completely open about hir reform school background while the rest explained that they had controlled what they told others about their past. The participants found that with time it had become easier to tell others about their backgrounds, but everyone had experiences of situations in which they wanted to conceal it. Some of them only talked about their past if they were asked, or only to people very special to them.

Perhaps I was a bit ashamed at first, for example I was going out [–] with this lovely X. I was X's first love and X's mum and dad were like really normal, you know, with high morals. X's mum was [academic professional] and dad was [respected professional] and y'know when you hope they won't find out. That you won't give away any clue about yourself before they have even met you. That's really the type of negative side that it has had I think. [–] It took ages, it took me ages before I told anyone [E: Yes]. We're really talking about over half a year here and then I told someone. And I tried to work out how I would tell X. I was really shitting myself, about what I would tell X so X would not lose interest in me.

(Interview)

The participant finally decided to be open about hir past. The relationship did not last, but in the interview the participant said that even though s/he used to be ashamed of hir past, s/he had decided not to hide it anymore. In Figure 9.5, the description of the participant has been illustrated with the position model. The position of being a former reform school student is reacted upon by significant others with prejudice, whereas for the participant the placement saved hem from drug addiction and school failure. This caused changes in hir behaviour: instead of

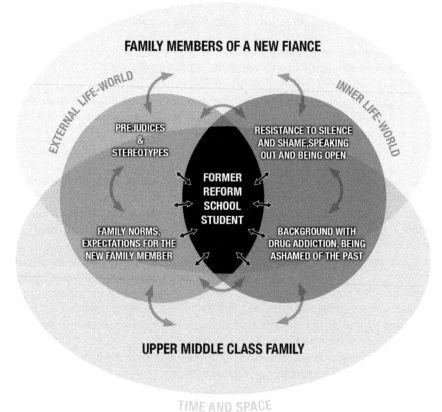

Figure 9.5 The position of a former reform school student in the system of structure, agency, and individual's life-world

silencing the past, s/he has chosen to be open about it. This was the most interesting result of the study: the negative position of a former reform school student was being actively reacted upon by these subjects themselves in the form of telling alternative stories, participating in a group that aims at developing the care given in the reform schools, and participating in this research, where the experiences of the young people have been studied.

When I asked about the significance of child welfare experiences, all participants felt that the events had had a significant impact on their life-world. A positive impact about it was, above all, the enabling of life opportunities, as the participants felt that their life before being taken into care was harmful and kept them from living a normal life. All participants had accepted the child welfare actions and felt that their experience of being taken into care was an important part of their own life story. They felt that the difficult experiences had given them self-assurance and confidence in their own survival. However, they did not have much confidence in the actions of social services, and the participants explained how they avoided social services as much as they could and would only resort to them if they were in extreme trouble, if then. The result of the research can be seen as a paradox as these young people had been provided the most intensive care that there is. Despite this, they felt they had been forced to manage and survive alone.

Discussion

In this study, I discovered that the children were affected by the multi-level societal reactions of their families, neighbourhoods, peer-groups, schools, and child welfare institutions, and that these reactions to a great extent defined the positions that were given to these children. The families of these children played a significant part, and made me ask whether the tendency of these young people to stray and commit offences, participate in substance use, and other norm-breaking behaviour, was a rational escape from the insecure and damaging relations of the families (Lemert, 1967, p. 48). The societal reactions of the other people did not support the children in these vulnerable situations, but left them coping on their own. By the time the children reached young adolescence, their insecurity and lack of trust became visible. They started to act out with disruptive behaviours that prompted negative societal reactions in the communities. In the school system, these young people were unable to meet the standards of a qualified student, and were thus dismissed. In their neighbourhoods, their actions resulted in conflicts with peers and contacts with the police. In the end, they were removed from their everyday communities.

In my earlier research, I have applied the position model to study the reasoning of social workers through child welfare documents in similar cases of young people. This side of the reality – the social worker's reasoning and decision-making processes – were not the focus of this research. This might be considered as a weakness of this analysis. In the child welfare documents, the shifts in the practices of social workers were affected by the multi-level changes in the resources of the social work agency, legislation, academic doctrines and networks of other professionals. In a very fundamental way, the reactions of the social workers and other agents were based on the idea of the humanity they were committed to (Pekkarinen, 2010). These shifts in reactions could be detected in both studies through the framework I applied: concentrating the focus of analysis on the societal reactions of different agents opened viewpoints and revealed external and internal mediators of the positions which would have not become visible if my focus had solely been on the behaviour of the child. However, at the level of the children's agency and experiences, the motives and working methods of social work remained a mystery, as their needs and opinions were repeatedly ignored. This is surprising, as child-centred methods have been at the core of Finnish social work since the beginning of the 1990s (e.g. Pösö, 2011) and the rights of children to participate have been emphasised in child welfare in particular.

We still rely on strong social images of delinquent youth and provide rigid lim-its for approved agency of children (James & James, 2001, pp. 212–214). These young people's behaviour was often pressured through the rigid boundaries of the situations they lived in. However, through empirical analysis I suggest that these young people were not passive victims of oppressing positions: they were indeed active agents and behaved accordingly. In many ways, the agency of these young people supported the position of a "defiant problem youth" or "reform school students". However, in light of the theory of societal reaction, I suggest that the behaviour which seemed irrational – such as committing offence after offence – seemed often to be a rational search for social recognition (Barry, 2006). The only relations that provided these young people social recognition were usually the peer groups, among which the breaking of the community norms was the actual norm. The eight young people researched had a clear, analytic, and honest way of perceiving their past situations, where they had only limited capacity to transform the social structures they were living in. Thus, they were actively trying to change the prejudices and stereotypes that are expressed toward the position of a reform school student, and thus transforming their past positions in the present.

Conclusion: Position model for analysing agency and structure

In this article, I described how a position model, constructed with the help of Bhaskar's texts, helps to organise the complex relationships between institutional and social structures and individuals' agency in a temporal context, and how we should more carefully perceive the individual's experiences of different positions. With the conceptual aid of Edwin M. Lemert's societal reaction theory, the arti-cle reveals how the social positions of eight former reform school students were shaped in the social and institutional contexts that they were present in, and how the young people have experienced these positions themselves. This empirical article also shows how social positions should not be analysed as passive aspects of role, or solely as objectively perceived problematic situations or contexts associated with normative expectations (see Archer, 1998, pp. 371–372), but as complicated situations in everyday life that are associated with not only roles of different agents and institutions, and normative expectations of different agents, but also with the individual's inner competences, expectations, norms, and courses of action. The article also reveals how people's self-understanding is affected by the labels they carry due to not only their personal histories but particularly due to the histories of the positions they are associated with in their social reality.

In this article, I described the way in which I have applied this position model developed on the basis of Roy Bhaskar's position – practice system, in the assess-ment of an empirical interview study with eight former reform school students. The model works particularly well in the assessment of individual cases, but by raising the abstraction level, the model could also be applied, for example, to the study of subcultures and other groups in certain positions. In this case, the exam-ined group's definitions of their own actions, norms and values can be applied to the part of the model that describes the inner life-world. The theoretical concepts linked to the model can be changed, but it is particularly well suited to the assessment of social interaction and social relationships. The model assists in guiding empirical attention toward the various mechanisms of social reality and the events that occur in the domain of the actual. It helps in taking the different structures, norms, values, reactions, relations, and agents into account, and aids in looking at the individual's inner processes as well. I believe it also has value in the practical tasks of social work in which an individual's position in a broader community or society as whole needs to be assessed.

Notes

1 The citations from the interviews have been made anonymous by removing or reconstructing information that might lead to identifying the participants. In addition, useless phrases such as "like" and "you know" have been removed as long as removing does not change the meaning of the sentence. The sexes of the participants have been neutralized by using the concepts s/he, hem, and hir.

[—] = a word or a part of the speech has been removed
[word] = a word added by the researcher that clarifies or replaces something in the text
E = researcher
P = participant in the interview

2 The postdoctoral research project has been funded by the Academy of Finland (267602/2013).
3 Reform schools are institutions in the Finnish child welfare system with a long history of institutional care among minors with disruptive behaviour, severe social problems, and offending. Of the currently existing reform schools, five are owned by the state and two are privately owned. Approximately 270 minors are annually placed in these institutions, which are located in rural areas in different parts of the country. In the field of child welfare services, the reform schools represent the most challenging form of care provided to the most challenging group of young people.

References

Archer, M. (1995) *Realist Social Theory: The Morphogenetic Approach*, Cambridge: Cambridge University Press.

Archer, M. (1998) Realism and Morphogenesis. In Bhaskar, R., Archer, M., Collier, A., Lawson, T., & Norrie, A. (eds.), *Critical Realism – Essential Readings*, London: Routledge, pp. 356–381.

Archer, M. S. (2000) *Being Human: The Problem of Agency*, Cambridge: Cambridge University Press.

Barry, M. (2006) *Youth Offending in Transition: The Search for Social Recognition*, London: Routledge.

Bhaskar, R. (1979) *The Possibility of Naturalism: A Philosophical Critique of the Contemporary Human Sciences*, Brighton: Harvester Press.

Bhaskar, R. (1986) *Scientific Realism & Human Emancipation*, London: Verso.

Bhaskar, R. (1993) *Dialectic: The Pulse of Freedom*, London: Verso.

Bhaskar, R. (1998) *The Possibility of Naturalism: A Philosophical Critique of the Contemporary Human Sciences* (3rd edn), Sussex: Harvester Press.

Garland, D. (2001) *The Culture of Control: Crime and Social Order in Contemporary Society*, Oxford: Oxford University Press.

Goffman, E. (1963) *Stigma: Notes on the Management of Spoiled Identity*, London: Penguin Books.

Harré, R. (2012) Positioning Theory: Moral Dimensions of Social-Cultural Psychology. In Valsiner, J. (ed.), *The Oxford Handbook of Culture and Psychology*, New York: Oxford University, pp. 191–206.

Harré, R. & van Langenhove, L. (eds.) (1999) *Positioning Theory*, Oxford: Blackwell Publisher.

James, A., & James, A. (2001) Tightening the net: Children, community, and control, *British Journal of Sociology*, 52(2), 211–228.

Kaidesoja, T. (2009) The Concept of Social Structure in Roy Bhaskar's Critical Realism. In Kaidesoja, T. (ed.), *Studies on Ontological and Methodological Foundations of Critical Realism in the Social Sciences*, Jyväskylä Studies in Education, Psychology and Social Research 376. Jyväskylä: University of Jyväskylä, www.academia.edu/4218954/The_Concept_of_Social_Structure_in_Roy_Bhaskars_Critical_Realism, 2 January, 2017.

Lemert, C., & Winter, M. F. (eds.) (2000) *Crime and Deviance: Essays and Innovations of Edwin M. Lemert*, Lanham, MD: Rowman & Littlefield Publishers.

Lemert, E. M. (1948) Some aspects of a general theory of sociopathic behavior, *Proceedings of the Pacific Sociological Society*, 16(1), 23–9.

Lemert, E. M. (1951) *Social Pathology: A Systematic Approach to the Theory of Sociopathic Behavior*, New York: McGraw-Hill.

Lemert, E. M. (1967) *Human Deviance, Social Problems & Social Control*, Englewood Cliffs, NJ: Prentice-Hall Sociology Series.

Lemert, E. M. (1974) Beyond mead: The societal reaction to deviance, *Social Problems*, 21(4), 457–468. doi:10.2307/799985.

Lemert, E. (2000) How We Got Where We Are: An Informal History of the Study of Deviance. In Lemert, C. & Winter, M. F. (eds.), *Crime and Deviance: Essays and Innovations of Edwin M. Lemert*, Lanham, MD: Rowman & Littlefield Publishers, pp. 66–74.

Muncie, J. (2004) *Youth and Crime* (2nd edn), London: Sage.

Pekkarinen, E. (2010) *Stadilaispojat, rikokset ja lastensuojelu: Viisi tapausta kuudelta vuosikymmeneltä [The Stadi-boys, Crimes and Child Welfare: Five Cases From Six Decades]*, Helsinki: Nuorisotutkimusverkosto & Nuorisotutkimusseura.

Pekkarinen, E. (2014) Positiomalli rakenteellisen sosiaalityön tukena [position model for structural social work]. In Pohjola, A., Laitnin, M., & Seppanen, M. (eds.), *Rakentellinen sosiaalityo [Structural Social Work]*, Kuopip: UNIpress, pp. 214–233.

Pekkarinen, E. (2017) *Koulukoti muutoksessa: Selvitys koulukotien asemasta ja tehavasta [Reform School in Change: Study on the Position and Tasks of Reform Schools]*, Helsinki: Nuorisotutkimusverkosto & Nuorisotutkimusseura.

Petrunik, M. (1980) The rise and fall of "labelling theory": The construction and destruction of a sociological strawman, *Canadian Journal of Sociology*, 5(3), 213–233.

Porpora, D. V. (1998) Four Concepts of Social Structure. In Bhaskar, R., Archer, M., Collier, A., Lawson, T., & Norrie, A. (eds.), *Critical Realism – Essential Readings*, London: Routledge, pp. 339–355.

Pösö, T. (2011) Combatting Child Abuse in Finland: From Family to Child-Centered Orientation. In Gilbert, N., Parton, N., & Skivenes, M. (eds.), *Child Protection Systems: International Trends and Orientations*, New York: Oxford University Press, pp. 112–130.

Pösö, T., & Huhtanen, R. (2016) Removals of Children in Finland: A Mix of Voluntary and Involuntary Decisions. In Burns, K., Pösö, T., & Skivenes, M. (eds.), *Child Welfare*

Removals by the State: A Cross-Country Analysis of Child Welfare Systems, New York: Oxford University Press, 18–39.

Seidman, I. (2013) *Interviewing as Qualitative Research: A Guide for Researchers in Education & the Social Sciences* (4th edn), New York: Teachers College Press.

Taylor, I., Walton, P., & Young, J. (1973) *The New Criminology: For a Social Theory of Deviance*, London: Routledge & Kegan Paul.

Part IV

10 Theory and practice as a dynamic relation

Monica Kjørstad and May-Britt Solem

The intention with this book is to introduce critical realism as ontology and as a metatheory. The aim is to explore critical realism as a theory of science that may contribute to a useful and realistic approach to research and practice for professionals who are working in different fields of social, welfare, and health work. It describes critical realism "in practice" by presenting examples of applications in four different empirical research projects. The presentations describe the normative and interdisciplinary components of critical realism and discuss how these dimensions are relevant and necessary for the development of ethical and value-based practices in welfare and health professional practices. We hope that the book will be relevant for professionals with a practice-oriented focus. In this concluding chapter, we wish to explore the relationship between theory and practice in the development of knowledge.

Entering this discussion, our own position is not conflationary; we are not simply trying to find a synthesis between theory and practice, but instead we wish to investigate this relationship from a dialectic and dynamic stance. This position raises the question: Where and when does knowledge appear? We will argue that knowledge emerges from the development of theories, from abstractions, *and* from practical work. A common example is the professional knowledge of a carpenter, a baker, an engineer, a nurse, or a social worker. An experienced practitioner has knowledge about how to handle a specific situation with his or her body, so to speak. Based on one's theoretical knowledge and practical experience, an excellent practitioner knows what to do in every specific situation using the art of making situational discriminations (Dreyfus & Dreyfus, 1986). This wisdom has been with us for a long time.

In Aristotelian language, this reasoning is understandable in the concept of *phrónesis*. Elaborating on this classic concept, Bent Flyvbjerg (2003) presented a way out of what he calls the "Science Wars" by developing a concept of social science based on a contemporary interpretation of the Aristotelian concept phrónesis (prudence or practical wisdom) (Flyvbjerg, 2003). Phrónesis goes beyond both analytical, scientific knowledge (episteme), and technical knowledge (*techne* – know how) and is commonly involved in social practice (Ibid.). Aristotle links phrónesis directly with political science. Prudence concerning the state has two aspects: one, which is controlling and directive, is legislative science. The other deals with particular circumstances and is practical and deliberative. Following this reasoning, Aristotle states that what is crucial for understanding and for praxis is what happens where the two now largely separate sides intersect, and that this point of intersection is the locus of appropriate phronetic activity (Flyvbjerg, 2003).

Present rhetoric

The relationship between the academic world and the professional social and welfare work practice is influenced by the growing interest in the need to provide research that scrutinises professional practice. Because significant public economic resources are allocated to the social sector, the public and policymakers are demanding *evidence-based knowledge* about the practice and the effects of social and welfare work. This may be partly motivated by the managerial potential of the concept. There is insufficient information about the effects and consequences of the methods and interventions of social work and there is increasing demand for systematic evaluation of social work practice (Kjørstad, 2008).

Despite the substantial public and scientific interest in evidence-based knowledge, there is no general agreement about the definition of the concept (Humphries, 2003; Shaw, 2005). At one extreme position, it is argued that the essence of evidence-based knowledge is that interventions must be founded on scientific evidence based on cause-and-effect explanations (Ekeland, 1999). At the other extreme, it is argued that evidence-based knowledge is based on *convincing arguments* (Marthinsen, 2004). A highly relevant perspective is presented by Humphries, who argued that evidence is seldom without ambiguity and policy and that practice is often not based on evidence, but on ideology and politics. In this way, the available evidence may be ignored (Humphries, 2003).

These arguments do not solely affect research methodology; they have a more general impact on the relationship between research and society as well (Kjørstad, 2008). Forty years ago, Robert Merton argued that all science is *in* society and that all science is formed *by* society (Merton & Storer, 1973). A similar view was later advocated by Davis Hess, who claimed that science and society are produced at the same time and intertwined and bound together in a seamless web. Separating the two is neither possible nor desirable (Hess, 1997). Scientific controversies may arise when internal and external conditions of scientific interests are in conflict and may strongly influence the priority of publicly financed research programs.

Practical knowledge and critical realism

Practical knowledge and everyday concepts have a special place within the critical realist perspective. The content of everyday knowledge makes up the immediate mechanisms behind the actions that build social phenomena. For that reason, everyday knowledge must be included within the focus of social science research (Danermark et al., 2002). The content of everyday knowledge belongs to "the raw material" that scientific knowledge must systematically include if theories in social science are to have validity (Ibid.). That means that concepts are not simply conceptions *about* or *within* society; they are often constituents of the social phenomenon itself that make up the field of research. This implies that the construction of social science concepts must be justified by the content of everyday knowledge and must be able to integrate that knowledge. At the same time, social science concepts must be able to transcend everyday concepts and be useful theoretically to provide clarification at a higher level (Ibid., p. 72). Theory plays a fundamental role in the research process and facts are seen as being *dependent* upon theory, but not *determined* by theory.

However, since social science concepts often are far removed from the experience that everyday knowledge is built upon, there will be a rivalry between everyday knowledge/common sense and scientific knowledge/concepts (Danermark et al., 2002). In social science, one is often in conflict with alternative experiences and concepts when trying to penetrate a level of reality that cannot directly be observed. Generative mechanisms can reveal this effort and occasionally challenge vital power relationships and social domination (Ibid.). Connecting to this line of thought, Sayer (1992; 2008) has argued that a great deal of our knowledge that is insufficient for prediction may be valuable for guidance. Any quest for certainty or "fixed correlations" between social variables is useless. Mechanisms produce "tendencies" and direct our attention toward seeking to understand and explain those tendencies (Archer et al., 1998; Sayer, 1992).

The practical fallacy

Referring to Sayer (1992; 2011), it follows that theorizing without reference to praxis and gained purely through contemplation or observation of the world is an "intellectual fallacy" (Sayer, 1992, p. 13). We may also argue that theory is a prerequisite for all forms of analytically based practice and a pathway to understand and explain phenomena in the world. When working with science and research, we need theories as prerequisites, giving direction to our methodology, as a premise or precondition. If not, we may be trapped in a "practical fallacy". However, no one theory can explain everything, and a realistic understanding of theories always includes an understanding of all theories' incompleteness. Nonetheless, theories provide a way of making sense and integral meaning of complexity and uncertainty.

A dialectical approach to the understanding of knowledge development

In the development of knowledge in social, welfare, and health work, the shortcomings of dichotomic thinking are apparent. Dialectic critical realism may be one method for overcoming formal dualism and reductionism (materialism-idealism, rationalism-empiricism, structure-agency, mind-body, theory-practice, positivism-constructivism) and makes it possible to transcend the opposites entailing a leap of the imagination to a higher level. Following this line of thought, one must transcend the dichotomies and the rhetorical phrases that are often encapsulated in the everyday life of many public institutions (Kjørstad, 2016 with reference to Bhaskar, 1986; 1993).

Referring to Alan Norrie (2010), Bhaskar's first phase of critical realism was an answer to the question of whether naturalism was possible, whereas the second (dialectic) phase was about the possibility of change, where Bhaskar developed a radically new and original theory of dialectics. It is about making a transcendental movement to overcome the most common dichotomies that are interwoven in our languages and embedded in all everyday practices, finding radically new knowledge. This transcendental movement is crucial for the possibility of change and the development of knowledge about human conditions. This might "answer" the question about the sources of new knowledge. Change-oriented understanding of the world is crucial to professional practices; consequently, this focus on change offers an illuminating viewpoint for social work research and practice. Dialectic thinking may uncover mechanisms that cause human problems and reveal how mechanisms and occurrences interact in different contexts. Another aspect of this transcendental movement is that it might help to think in an interdisciplinary manner to understand the grand societal challenges of our time.

The essence of dialectic methods is to raise questions and find answers, evidence and counter-evidence, arguments and counter-arguments. This is relevant with respect to the search for generative mechanisms that cause social and societal problems, which are at the core of critical realism. Dialectic exercising and thinking may uncover mechanisms that cause human problems and reveal how mechanisms and occurrences interact in different contexts (Kjørstad, 2016). The intention is to find the meaning of constructs and to investigate practice *in depth* in order to understand social problems and social interventions on a deeper level than the empirical, observational level (Houston, 2001).

The distinction that Bhaskar made on this point is crucial. The aim is not to find some conflationary position or statement, but by real transcendence of the dichotomies, to search for *emerging mechanisms* that may point out new understandings of reality and, in some lucky moments, an integral understanding and insights that may lead to new knowledge.

Explicating presuppositions

The transcendental argument is part of this reasoning. Such an argument asks what must be the case for some feature of our experience to be possible – what must the world be like for some social practice to be possible? The retroductive argument then asks what would, if it were real, bring about, produce, cause, or explain a phenomenon. Following this line of thought, according to Bhaskar, retroduction is "the imaginative activity in science by which the scientist thinks up causes and generative mechanisms which, if they were real, would explain the phenomenon in question" (Bhaskar, 2016, p. 3).

Immanent critique

Immanent critique is another essential part of the method of critical realist philosophy (Bhaskar, 2016, p. 2). Bhaskar argues that criticism of an idea or a system should be internal, that is, involve something intrinsic to what is being criticized (Bhaskar, 2016, p. 3). Immanent critique might identify theory/practice inconsistencies, showing that the position being disputed involves a claim or analysis that would undermine the point, values, or substance of the position; so that it undermines or "deconstructs" itself (Bhaskar, 2016, p. 3). In this exercise, it is crucial to also include what one's opponents believe. This demonstrates the need for research about knowledge in your own "circles" and formulate critical questions about the hegemony of one's own discipline. What is taken for granted should be challenged.

Applied critical realism

The strength of critical realism is that it is applicable. Sceptics argue that critical realism is theoretically consistent and coherent, while the methodology and application of critical realism is less developed. Roy Bhaskar sometimes explained 'practical', or applied, critical realism as *organic* critical realism. It is important to remember that critical realist research is characterised by the *primacy of ontology* in the research process, in contrast to positivism and social constructivism where the epistemology is primary (Bhaskar, 2016, p. 79).

Accordingly, the interests of critical realists in empirical research are exploratory. It puts explanation in the first place – prediction is secondary. The primary focus is on structures and mechanisms, not regularities and patterns of events (Bhaskar, 2016, p. 79). Because social phenomena occur in open systems, characterised by complexity and emergence, one may not talk about predictability, but of tendencies.

Interdisciplinarity as necessity

The multiplicity of causes, mechanisms, and theories "in itself licence the transition to multidisciplinarity" (Bhaskar, 2016, p. 16). For that the emergence of levels are needed, which means that some of the mechanisms in an applied or concrete explanation are ontologically distinct and irreducible to the more basic ones. Bhaskar is pointing out that this gives us *multidisciplinarity* – however, that is not yet *interdisciplinarity*. For interdisciplinarity to become, one needs non-additive relations between distinct levels, or the emergence of outcomes. The emergence of the mechanisms themselves produce intradisciplinarity (Bhaskar, 2016, p. 15). "The *holy trinity of interdisciplinarity research* and inter-professional cooperation quickly follows: this involves metatheoretical unity, methodological specificity and substantive theoretical pluralism and tolerance" (Bhaskar, 2016, p. 16).

The contributions of this book are all about issues that are at the core of critical realism. The legitimacy of norms and values in social science research is underscored in the article by Andrew Sayer. In his contribution, Berth Daner-mark is arguing for the necessity of interdisciplinary approaches to handle societal problems of great complexity. Stan Houston and Lorna Montgomery demonstrate the use of a dialectic method, discussing the relevance of critical realism in prob-lem-based learning in education. The empirical contributions by Harry Lunabba, Elina Pekkarinen, May-Britt Solem, and Monica Kjørstad are all examples of the applicability of critical realism to empirical research in the different fields of social science.

What is common for all the contributions in the book is that *seriousness* is one of the distinctive features of critical realism. We think it would be appropriate to close the book with these encouraging words from Roy Bhaskar:

> What critical realism would like to do, then, is produce a serious philosophy that we can act on, and one moreover that is relevant to the pressing chal-lenges we face and that ideally at least can illuminate a way forward (telling us something new).
>
> (Bhaskar, 2016, p. 2)

References

Archer, M. S., Bhaskar, R., Collier, A., Lawson, T., Norrie, A., Bhaskar, R., Collier, A., Law-son, T., & Norrie, A. (1998) *Critical Realism: Essential Readings*, London: Routledge.

Bhaskar, R. (1986) *Scientific Realism & Human Emancipation*, London: Verso.

Bhaskar, R. (1993) *Dialectic: The Pulse of Freedom*, London: Verso.

Bhaskar, R. Edited with a preface by Mervyn Hartwig (2016) *Enlightened Common Sense: The Philosophy of Critical Realism*, London: Routledge.

Danermark, B., Ekström, M., Jakobsen, L., & Karlsson, J. C. (2002) *Explaining Society: Critical Realism in the Social Sciences*, London: Routledge.

Dreyfus, H. L., & Dreyfus, S. E. (1986) *Mind Over Machine: The Power of Human Intui-tion and Expertise in the Era of the Computer*, New York: The Free Press & MacMillan.

Ekeland, T. J. (1999) Evidensbasert behandling: Kvalitetssikring eller instrumentalistisk Mistak [Evidence-based therapy: An assurance for quality, or an instrumental failure], *Tidskrift for Norsk Psykologforening*, 36(11), 1036–1047.

Flyvbjerg, B. (2003) *Making Social Science Matter*, Cambridge: Cambridge University Press.

Hess, D. J. (1997) *Science Studies: An Advanced Introduction*, New York: New York Uni-versity Press.

Houston, S. (2001) Beyond social constructionism: Critical realism and social work, *Brit-ish Journal of Social Work*, 31, 845–861.

Humphries, B. (2003) What else counts as evidence in evidence-based social work? *Social Work Education*, 22(1), 81–91.

Kjørstad, M. (2008) Et kritisk, realistisk perspektiv på sosialt arbeid i forvaltningen: En studie av sosialarbeideres iverksetting av arbeidslinjen i norsk sosialpolitikk [A Critical Realist Perspective on Social Work in the Public Services: A Study of Social Work-ers' Implementation of a Workfare Policy in Norway], Doktoravhandlinger ved NTNU 2008: 308, Norges teknisk-naturvitenskapelige universitet (NTNU).

Kjørstad, M. (2016) Leadership as Ethical Agency in the Social Welfare Services -Need for Re-Humanisation? A Critical Realist Perspective. *Work in Progress. Paper presented at the 19th Annual Conference of Critical Realism*, University of Cardiff, Cardiff business school, 19–22 July.

Marthinsen, E. (2004) "Evidensbasert": Praksis og Ideologi [Evidence-based: Practice and ideology], *Nordisk Sosialt Arbeid*, 24(4), 290–302.

Merton, R. K., & Storer, N. W. (1973) *The Sociology of Science: Theoretical and Empirical Investigations*, Chicago, IL: The University of Chicago Press.

Norrie, A. (2010) *Dialectic and Difference: Dialectical Critical Realism and the Grounds of Justice*, London: Routledge.

Sayer, A. (1992) *Method in Social Science: A Realist Approach*, London: Routledge.

Sayer, A. (2008) *Realism and Social Science*, London: Sage.

Sayer, A. (2011) *Why Things Matter to People: Social Science, Values and Ethical Life*, Cambridge: Cambridge University Press.

Shaw, I. (2005) Practitioner research: Evidence or critique, *British Journal of Social Work*, 35(8), 1231–1248.

Index

Note: Page numbers in italic indicate figures.

abductive analyses 111
abductive redescription/
    recontextualisation 46
absence, notion (usage) 69–70
absenting, impact 64
acid test 49–50
action: external conditions 123–4; external
    definitions 124; inner conditions 125;
    inner definitions 125
activation (workfare rhetoric) 80
actual domain 93
agency: analysis, position model (usage)
    138–9; child vulnerability, position *128*;
    defiant/problem youth position *132*;
    former reform school student position
    136; reform school student position
    134; structure, dialectic relation 85;
    system *124*
agents, social interactions 48
applied critical realism, usage 149
Archer, Margaret 99
articulating activities 85
ATLAS analysis 126
attachment, mechanism 61
attunement, concept 100–1
autonomic agent, freedom 120
autonomic nervous system, structure 42

Bhaskar, Roy 10, 15–16, 57, 64, 120, 123,
    138, 150; question 17
biological determinism 26
biological mechanisms 48
biopsychosocial model 48
black-box approach 85–6
Bowlby, John 61
Bronfenbrenner, Urie 48
bureaucratic ethics 82

CAIMeR theory, usage 59
capability approach 30–1
care: ethic 24; importance 32–3
causality, change 60, 63–5
cause-and-effect explanations 85
cause-and-effect models 7
causes, multiplicity 149
child abuse, social problem (Sweden) 50
child welfare: agency/structure (analysis),
    position model (usage) 138–9; data/
    method 126–7; discussion 137–8;
    early adolescence, positions 129–31;
    early childhood, positions 127–9;
    experiences, significance 136–7;
    former reform school student, position
    136; interventions, young people
    positions/experiences (impact) 127–37;
    position-practice system 120–1; reform
    school student, position 131–7, *134*;
    societal reaction, theory 121–3; study,
    research questions 119–20; study,
    theoretical framework 119–20; young
    people, positions 118
classroom structures, focus 94–7
closed conditions 16
closed systems, dichotomy 51
collectivism 101
commodification, function 61
competence, dignity (association) 32
complexity theory 69
confidence 127
consciousness, expansion 46
constructivism 147
Context-Mechanism-Outcome
    (C-M-O) configuration 77, *83*;
    project adaptation 82
context-sensitive analyses, CR support 107

change 50; child vulnerability, position *128*; system, defiant/problem youth position *132*; system, former reform school student position *136*; system, reform school student position *134*
structure-mechanisms-event 42–3
subjective mechanisms 99
survey instruments, usage 114–15
systemic practices 8

theory: building, logic 46; metatheory, necessity/autonomy 53; multiplicity 149
theory/practice: dynamic relation 145; fallacy 147–8; immanent critique 149; interdisciplinarity, necessity 149–50; presuppositions 148–9; rhetoric 146–7
thick ethical descriptions 28
thin ethical concepts 28
things-as-we-see-them 62
things-in-themselves 62
totality 65, 68
transcendental question, initiation 68–9
Transformational Model of Social Activity (TMSA) 10, 120–1; usage 119
transformative function 38–9
transformative praxis 65
transitive dimensions 53, 62

unconscious, symbolic contents 46
under labourer, action 57
universalism: conventionalism, contrast 30; values, relationship 29–31

values: critical realism perspective 31; dichotomization, absurdity 29; misunderstanding 28–29; universalism, relationship 29–31; values-informed social work research 59

welfare dependency 83
welfare work: intellectual fallacy, relationship 5–6; normative position 8–9; social politics, dynamics (understanding) 77; understanding 3
work, precondition 43–4
workfare: concepts 80; design 82–3; ethical implications 80–1; project 81–4; reciprocity, generative mechanism 83–4; social worker practice 81
world, change-oriented understanding 148

young masculinities (ethnographic research), critical realism/domain theory (implementation) 90

For Product Safety Concerns and Information please contact our EU
representative GPSR@taylorandfrancis.com
Taylor & Francis Verlag GmbH, Kaufingerstraße 24, 80331 München, Germany